Foundations of Psychiatric Mental Health Nursing

Third Edition

Elizabeth M. Varcarolis, R.N., M.A.

Professor Emeritus
Borough of Manhattan Community College
New York, NY

Associate Fellow
Albert Ellis Institute for Rational Emotive Behavioral Therapy (REBT)
New York, NY

W.B. SAUNDERS COMPANY
A Harcourt Health Sciences Company
St. Louis   Philadelphia   London   Sydney   Toronto

W.B. SAUNDERS COMPANY

A *Harcourt Health Sciences Company*

The Curtis Center
Independence Square West
Philadelphia, Pennsylvania 19106

DRUG NOTICE

Psychiatric Nursing is an ever-changing field. Standard safety precautions must be followed, but as new research and clinical experience broaden our knowledge, changes in treatment and drug therapy become necessary or appropriate. Readers are advised to check the product information currently provided by the manufacturer of each drug to be administered to verify the recommended dose, the method and duration of administration, and contraindications. It is the responsibility of the treating physician relying on experience and knowledge of the patient to determine dosages and the best treatment for the patient. Neither the Publisher nor the editor assumes any responsibility for any injury and/or damage to persons or property.

The Publisher

Clinical Companion for
FOUNDATIONS OF PSYCHIATRIC
MENTAL HEALTH NURSING, third edition   ISBN 0-7216-7734-7

Copyright © 1998 by W.B. Saunders Company

All rights reserved. No part of this publication may be reproduced or transmitted in any form or by any means, electronic or mechanical, including photocopy, recording, or any information storage and retrieval system, without permission in writing from the publisher.

Printed in the United States of America.

Last digit is the print number: 9   8   7   6   5   4   3   2

PREFACE

Welcome to your psychiatric nursing experience. This clinical guide is a quick reference for many of the common phenomena that you will encounter in psychiatric nursing.

The included assessment data, tools, and guidelines are designed to help you identify specific behaviors. The tools in this guide will help you assess levels of anxiety and identify risk factors associated with potential for suicide, depression, and violence.

The nursing guidelines in the *Clinical Companion* give you a frame of reference for key intervention strategies and areas of concerns. Understanding intervention strategies for phenomena such as depression, mania, delusions, hallucinations, paranoia, anxiety, manipulation, and hostility, among others, is a key focus of your psychiatric nursing education.

Psychopharmacotherapy is key in management of many of the biologically-based mental disorders such as the mood disorders and schizophrenia. This guide provides a quick reference for some of the more common medications, including dosages commonly used for specific disorders and their side and toxic effects. Each group of medications includes guides for client and family teaching, which is one of the most important nursing tasks in our effort to help empower and inform our client population.

The appendices in this *Clinical Companion* also include helpful information: The Mini-Mental State Examination, a selected list of self-help and support groups that may be appropriate for some of your clients, and detailed information about several common medications. I hope you find this a useful clinical reference during your psychiatric nursing experience.

Best of luck!

Elizabeth Varcarolis

CONTENTS

Part I: Mood Disorders	**1**
Depression	2
Assessing for Depression	2
Psychopharmacology for Depression	5
Client and Family Teaching: Tricyclics	8
Client and Family Teaching: MAOIs	11
Client and Family Teaching: SSRIs	12
Mania	13
Assessing for Mania	13
Psychopharmacology for Mania	15
Client and Family Teaching: Lithium	16
Part II: Psychotic Disorders	**18**
Schizophrenia	19
Assessing for Hallucinations	19
Assessing for Delusions	21
Assessing for Paranoia	22
Psychopharmacology for Schizophrenia	24
Client and Family Teaching: Schizophrenia	27
Part III: Anxiety Disorders	**29**
Anxiety	30
Assessing for Anxiety	30
Psychopharmacology for Anxiety	34
Client and Family Teaching: Antianxiety Medications	36
Part IV: Clinical Behaviors Requiring Intervention	**37**
Suicide	38
Violence	42
Manipulation	46
Appendices	**49**
Appendix A: The Mini-Mental State Examination	50
Appendix B: Selected Self-Help and Support Groups	51
Appendix C: Selected Prototypical Medications	53
References	**75**

PART I

MOOD DISORDERS

DEPRESSION

Assessing for Depression

History

The following questions are intended as guidelines for obtaining a client's history when you assess for depression.

- Does client have a personal or family history of a mood disorder?
- Does client have a substance abuse or alcohol problem?
- Does client have a personality disorder (e.g., borderline) or eating disorder?
- Has client had a recent bereavement (loss)?
- Does client have an acute or chronic medical condition?

Presenting Symptoms

- Depressed mood (or irritability in children or adolescents)
- Diminished interest in or pleasure in most or all activities
- Alterations in eating, sleeping, activity level (fatigue), and libido
- Feelings of worthlessness or guilt
- Difficulty with concentration, memory, and making decisions
- Recurrent thoughts of death and/or self-harm

Assessment Guidelines

Use Zung's Self-Rating Depression Scale, shown in Table 1, to assess patient depression.

TABLE 1: ZUNG'S SELF-RATING DEPRESSION SCALE*

	None or Little of the Time	Some of the Time	A Good Part of the Time	Most or All of the Time
1. I feel downhearted, blue, and sad.	1	2	3	4
2. Morning is when I feel the best.	4	3	2	1
3. I have crying spells or feel like it.	1	2	3	4
4. I have trouble sleeping through the night.	1	2	3	4
5. I eat as much as I used to.	4	3	2	1
6. I enjoy looking at, talking to, and being with attractive women/men.	4	3	2	1
7. I notice that I am losing weight.	1	2	3	4
8. I have trouble with constipation.	1	2	3	4
9. My heart beats faster than usual.	1	2	3	4
10. I get tired for no reason.	1	2	3	4
11. My mind is as clear as it used to be.	4	3	2	1
12. I find it easy to do the things I used to do.	4	3	2	1
13. I am restless and can't keep still.	1	2	3	4
14. I feel hopeful about the future.	4	3	2	1
15. I am more irritable than usual.	1	2	3	4
16. I find it easy to make decisions.	4	3	2	1
17. I feel that I am useful and needed.	4	3	2	1
18. My life is pretty full.	4	3	2	1
19. I feel that others would be better off if I were dead.	1	2	3	4
20. I still enjoy the things I used to do.	4	3	2	1

*A raw score of 50 or above is associated with depression requiring hospital treatment.
From Zung, W.K. (1965). A self-rating depression scale. Archives of General Psychiatry, 12:63. Copyright 1965, American Medical Association.

Sample Questions

To obtain further information about a client's mental status, ask the client the following questions, adapting them to the current situation.

- How is your general health? Has it changed recently?
- How is your sleep/bowels/libido/appetite? Have they changed recently?
- When you get sad or down, how long does it last?
- Do you find yourself avoiding people?
- Do you go out less than you used to?
- Are you hard on yourself? Have you been harder on yourself lately?
- What do you see for yourself in the future?
- When people get depressed, they sometimes think of dying. Have you had thoughts like this?
- Have you thought of hurting yourself?

Guidelines for Nursing Interventions

The following guidelines provide a basis for nursing interventions for the depressed client.

1. A sound physical and neurological exam helps to determine if the depression is primary or secondary to another disorder. Depression can be secondary to a host of medical or other psychiatric disorders. Essentially, the team needs to evaluate whether:
   a. The client is psychotic.
   b. The client has taken drugs or alcohol.
   c. There are medical conditions as causative factors.
2. Always evaluate the client's risk of harm to self or others. Overt hostility is highly correlated with suicide. (See "Assessing Potential for Suicide" in Part IV of this guide.)
3. Try to convey caring, empathy, understanding, and optimism. *The installation of hope is a key tool for recovery.*

4. Enhance the person's sense of self by highlighting strengths and past accomplishments.
5. Whether in the hospital or in the community:
   a. Assess the person's needs for self-care and offer support when appropriate.
   b. Monitor and intervene to help maintain adequate nutrition, hydration, and elimination.
   c. Monitor and intervene to help provide an adequate balance of rest, sleep, and activity.
   d. Involve client's support system; find appropriate supports in the community for client and family members.
6. Countering the dysfunctional attitude or learned helplessness often seen with depressed people requires cognitive therapy or other sociotherapeutic and psychotherapeutic interventions.
7. Primary depression is a disease that responds well to psychopharmacology. Be sure both client and family understand the nature of the disease and have written information about the specific medications client is taking. *Client teaching is vital.*
8. Combined psychopharmacotherapy and psychotherapy has been found to be more effective in treating major depression and in delaying the return of symptoms than either treatment alone (Slaby 1994).
9. Successful management of a depressive episode entails compliance with medication provided over the course of months and sometimes years.

Psychopharmacology for Depression

This section provides guidelines for adult dosages of antidepressants and describes side and toxic effects of these drugs. This section also lists important information to be given to client and client's family regarding the various medications.

TABLE 2: ADULT DOSAGES FOR ANTIDEPRESSANTS*

Generic Name (Trade Name)	Initial Dose*† (mg/Day)	Dose After 4–8 Weeks* (mg/Day)	Maximum* Dose (mg/Day)
Tricyclic Antidepressants (TCAs)			
Amitryptyline (Elavil, Endep)	50–150	100–200	300
Desipramine (Norpramin, Pertofrane)	50–150	75–200	300
Doxepin (Adapin, Sinequan)	50–150	100–200	300
Imipramine (Tofranil)	50–150	100–200	300
Nortriptyline (Aventyl, Pamelor)	25–100	75–150	150
Protriptyline (Vivactil)	10–40	15–40	60
Trimipramine (Surmontil)	50–150	75–250	250
Monoamine Oxidase Inhibitors (MAOIs)			
Isocarboxazid (Marplan)	20–30	20–30	30
Phenelzine (Nardil)	45–75	45–75	75
Tranylcypromine (Parnate)	20–30	20–30	30
Selective Serotonin Reuptake Inhibitors (SSRIs)			
Fluoxetine (Prozac)	20	20–40	80
Fluvoxamine (Floxyfral)*	50–100	50–300	300
Paroxetine (Paxil)	20	20–50	50
Sertraline (Zoloft)*	50	50–200	200
Selective Serotonin/Norepinephrine Reuptake Inhibitors (SSNRIs)			
Venlafaxine (Effexor)	75	75–225	375
Nefazodone (Serzone)	200	300–600	600
Atypical Antidepressants			
Amoxapine (Asendin)	50–150	200–300	400
Bupropion (Wellbutrin)	200	225–450	450
Maprotiline (Ludiomil)	50–150	100–150	225
Trazodone (Desyrel)	150	150–200	400–600

Adapted from Lehne, R.A., et al. (1994). *Pharmacology of Nursing*, 2nd ed. Philadelphia: W.B. Saunders; Robinson, D.S., et al. (1996). Therapeutic range of nefazodone in the treatment of depression. *Journal of Clinical Psychiatry*, 57(2):6–9.

*Doses listed are total daily doses. Depending on the drug and patient, the total dose may be given in a single dose or in divided doses. Doses higher than these may be needed for some clients with severe depression.
†Investigational agent.

TABLE 3: SIDE AND TOXIC EFFECTS OF TRICYCLICS

Phenomena	Comments
Anticholinergic Effects	
1. Dry mouth, blurred vision, postural hypotension, dry eyes, photophobia, nasal congestion	1. Most side effects are not serious and are transitory (1–2 weeks). For people with orthostatic hypotension, nortriptyline may be a good alternative.
2. Urinary retention and severe constipation	2. Bethanechol, 10–25 mg tid or tid-qid, may help urinary retention. Both urinary retention and severe constipation need immediate medical attention. Check for fecal impaction.
Cardiac Effects	
Note: *All patients should be checked for TCA-cardiac interactions before starting a TCA therapy.*	
1. Low blood pressure (hypotension with dizziness)	1a. Check blood pressure with client lying and standing.
	1b. Instruct client to rise slowly and hang onto objects.
	1c. Instruct client to use support hose.
	1d. Have physician change the TCA.
	1e. Occurs with greater frequency in patients with cardiac conditions.
	1f. Protect clients, especially elderly clients, against falls.
2. Tachycardia and arrhythmias	2. Use TCAs with caution in clients with cardiac conditions and in the elderly.
3. Cardiac ECG changes	3. TCAs are fatal in clients with second-degree and third-degree heart block.
4. Heart failure	4. Use with caution. Monitor client's vital signs regularly.
Central Nervous System Responses	
1. Sedation (especially during the first two weeks)	1. Have physician prescribe a less sedating TCA and give full dose at bedtime.

(Continued on next page)

TABLE 3, CONTINUED

Phenomena	Comments
Central Nervous System Responses, continued	
2. Delirium (in high doses)	2. Withhold further doses of the drug and contact the physician immediately.
3. Memory impairment (especially in the elderly)	3. Evaluate changes in status of client's memory.
4. Seizures (with maprotiline)	4. Most seizures reported for maprotiline result from administration of high doses.
5. "Spaciness," depersonalization	5. Increase drug dose more slowly or switch the TCA.
6. Tremors	6. Lower the dose. Physician may prescribe propranolol.
Endocrine and Sexual Effects	
1. Decreased or increased libido	1. Have physician evaluate; may change to another TCA.
2. Priapism (trazodone)	2. Medical intervention is crucial within 4–6 hours to maintain sexual ability.
3. Breast enlargement in women and men	3. Physician may try an alternative drug if this effect causes embarrassment (men/women).
4. Appetite stimulation	4. Weight gain can be a problem.

Data from Maxmen, J.S. and Ward, N.G. (1995). *Psychotropic drugs: Fast facts*, 2nd ed. New York: W.W. Norton; Preston, J., and Johnson, J. (1995). *Clinical psychopharmacology made ridiculously simple*. Miami, FL: Medmaster; Schatzberg, A.F., and Cole, J.O. (1991). *Manual of clinical psychopharmacology*, 2nd ed. Washington, DC: American Psychiatric Press.

ECG, electrocardiographic; TCA, tricyclic antidepressant; bid, twice a day; tid, three times a day; qid, four times a day.

Client and Family Teaching: Tricyclics

- Explain that mood elevation may take 7–28 days; it may take 6–8 weeks for full effect to take place and major symptoms to subside.
- Have family reinforce this frequently to client. Depressed people have trouble remembering and respond to ongoing reassurance.
- Reassure client that drowsiness, dizziness, and hypotension usually subside after the first few weeks.
- When client first begins taking TCAs, caution client to be careful working around machines, driving cars, or crossing streets due to possible altered reflexes, drowsiness, or dizziness.

- Explain to client why it is important to avoid alcohol; it can block effects of antidepressants.
- Teach client to take full dose at bedtime if possible to reduce the experience of side effects during the day.
- If client forgets the bedtime dose (or the once-a-day dose), client should take the dose within 3 hours; otherwise client should wait for the next day. Client should not double the dose.
- Suddenly stopping TCAs can cause nausea, altered heartbeat, nightmares, and cold sweats in 2–4 days. If these symptoms appear, client should call the physician or take one dose of the TCA until the physician can be contacted.

TABLE 4: SIDE AND TOXIC EFFECTS OF MAOIS

Side Effects	Comments
• Hypotension	Hypotension is the most critical side effect (10%); the elderly especially may sustain injuries from it.
• Sedation, weakness, fatigue • Insomnia • Changes in cardiac rhythm • Muscle cramps • Anorgasmia or sexual impotence • Urinary hesitancy or constipation • Weight gain	

Toxic Effects	Comments

Hypertensive crisis *
• Severe headache
• Stiff, sore neck
• Flushing; cold, clammy skin
• Tachycardia
• Severe nosebleeds, dilated pupils
• Chest pains, stroke, coma, death
• Nausea and vomiting
	1. Client should go to local emergency department immediately—blood pressure should be checked.
	2. Client may receive one of the following to lower blood pressure:
	  • Intravenous phentolamine (Regitine)
	  • Oral chlorpromazine
	  • Nifedipine (calcium channel blocker) 10 mg every hour IV until relief occurs (1–2 doses)

*Related to interaction with foods and cold medications.

TABLE 5: FOODS THAT CAN INTERACT WITH MAOIs

Foods That Contain Tyramine

Category	Unsafe Foods (High Tyramine Content)	Safe Foods (Little or No Tyramine)
Vegetables	Avocados, especially if overripe; fermented bean curd; fermented soybean; soybean paste, sauerkraut	Most vegetables
Fruits	Figs, especially if overripe; bananas, in large amounts	Most fruits
Meats	Meats that are fermented, smoked, or otherwise aged; spoiled meats; beef and chicken liver, unless very fresh	Meats that are known to be fresh (exercise caution in restaurants; meat may not be fresh)
Sausages	Fermented varieties; bologna, pepperoni, others	Nonfermented varieties
Fish	Dried, pickled, or cured fish; fish that is fermented, smoked, or otherwise aged; spoiled fish	Fish that is known to be fresh; vacuum-packed fish, if eaten promptly or refrigerated only briefly after opening
Milk, milk products	Practically all cheeses	Milk, yogurt, cottage cheese, cream cheese
Yeast	Yeast extract (e.g., Marmite, Bovril)	Baked goods that contain yeast
Beer, wine	Some imported beers, Chianti	Major domestic brands of beer; most wines
Other foods	Protein dietary supplements; soups (may contain protein extract); shrimp paste; soy sauce	

Foods That Contain Other Vasopressors

Food	Comments
Chocolate	Contains phenylethylamine, a pressor agent; large amounts can cause reaction.
Fava beans	Contain dopamine, a pressor agent; reactions are most likely with overripe beans.
Ginseng	Headache, tremulousness, and manic-like reactions have occurred.
Caffeine	Caffeine is a weak pressor agent; large amounts may cause a reaction.

From Lehne, R.A., et al. (1994). *Pharmacology for nursing*, 2nd ed. Philadelphia: W.B. Saunders.

TABLE 6: DRUGS THAT CAN INTERACT WITH MAOIs

- Over-the-counter medications for colds, allergies, or congestion (any product containing ephedrine, phenylephrine hydrochloride, or phenylpropanolamine)
- Tricyclic antidepressants (imipramine, amitriptyline)
- Narcotics
- Antihypertensives (methyldopa, guanethidine, reserpine)
- Amine precursors (levodopa, L-tryptophan)
- Sedatives (alcohol, barbiturates, benzodiazepines)
- General anesthetics
- Stimulants (amphetamines, cocaine)

Client and Family Teaching: MAOIs

- Teach client to avoid certain foods and all medications (especially cold remedies) unless prescribed by and discussed with physician.
- Give client a wallet card describing the MAOI regimen. (Parke-Davis will supply them if contacted at 1-800-223-6432.)
- Instruct client to avoid Chinese restaurants (sherry, brewer's yeast, and other products may be used.
- Instruct client to go to the emergency department right away if client has a severe headache.
- Instruct client to have blood pressure monitored during first 6 weeks of treatment (for both hypotensive and hypertensive effects).
- Explain to client the need to maintain dietary and drug restrictions for 14 days after stopping the MAOI.

TABLE 7: SIDE AND TOXIC EFFECTS OF SSRIs

Note: *Do not administer SSRIs to patients who are taking MAOIs. The drug interaction can result in serious or fatal reactions.*

Side Effects	Comments
1. Rash or allergic reaction	1. Discontinue drug; ask physician about treatment with antihistamines or steroids.
2. Anxiety, nervousness, insomnia	2. Discontinue the drug.

(Continued on next page)

TABLE 7, CONTINUED

3. Anorexia, weight loss, nausea,	3. Particularly common in underweight, depressed clients. If significant weight loss occurs, ask physician about changing to a different drug.
4. Tremors, sweating, dizziness, lightheadedness	4. Most of the effects listed in 4, 5, and 6 are transient and disappear when drug is discontinued.
5. Drowsiness and fatigue	5. SSRIs can affect cognitive motor ability.
6. Decreased or altered libido.	6. If change in libido becomes a problem for client, ask doctor about changing the drug.

Client and Family Teaching: SSRIs

- SSRIs may cause sexual dysfunction or lack of sex drive. Inform physician.
- SSRIs may cause insomnia, anxiety, and nervousness. Inform physician.
- SSRIs may interact with other medications. Be sure physician knows other medications client is taking (digoxin, warfarin). SSRIs should not be taken within 14 days of the last dose of an MAOI.
- Do not take any over-the-counter drugs without first notifying the physician.
- Common side effects include fatigue, nausea, diarrhea, dry mouth, dizziness, tremor, fatigue, and sexual dysfunction or lack of sex drive.
- Because of the potential for drowsiness and dizziness, client should not drive or operate machinery until these side effects are ruled out.
- Explain to client why it is necessary to avoid alcohol.
- Client should have liver and renal function tests performed and blood counts checked periodically.
- Teach client not to discontinue the medication abruptly. If side effects become bothersome, client should ask physician about

changing to a different drug, but be aware that the medication will have to be phased out over a period of time.

Report any of the following symptoms to physician immediately:

- Rash or hives
- Sore throat
- Fever, malaise
- Unusual bleeding
- Severe headache
- Rapid heart rate
- Difficulty urinating
- Anorexia/weight loss
- Initiation of hyperactive behavior

MANIA

Assessing for Mania

History

The following questions are intended as guidelines for obtaining a client's history when you assess for mania.

- Does client have a personal or family history of a bipolar illness?
- Has client had periods of elated or depressed moods in the past?
- Is client on any mood-altering drugs?
- Have all other medical and mental disorders been ruled out?

Presenting Symptoms

- Periods of hyperactivity (pacing, restlessness, speeding up)
- Overconfident, exaggerated view of own abilities
- Decreased need for sleep, no acknowledgment of fatigue
- Poor social judgment, engaging in reckless or self-destructive activities (foolish business ventures, sexual indiscretions, buying sprees)
- Rapid-fire or pressured speech; loud, garrulous, rhyming, punning
- Brief attention span, easily distractible, flights of ideas, loosened associations, delusions
- Expansive, irritable, or paranoid behaviors
- Impatient, uncooperative, abusive, obscene, manipulative

Assessment Guidelines

Use the following guidelines to assess a client for mania.

- Assess danger to self or others. Manic clients can exhaust themselves to the point of death. Clients may not eat or sleep for days at a time.
- Clients may give away all of their money or possessions; controls may need to be introduced to protect them from bankruptcy.
- Assess need for hospitalization to safeguard and stabilize client.
- Assess client's and family's understanding of bipolar disorder and the medications used to treat it.

Sample Questions

- Was there ever a time when you . . .
  - talked too much and couldn't stop?
  - started things you couldn't finish?
  - were too happy without any reason?
  - did without sleep or much food for a day or two?
  - spent money recklessly, spent money you didn't have, or made extravagant gifts?
- Have you ever found yourself pacing or moving and couldn't stop?
- Was there ever a time you couldn't stop your mind from racing?
- Was there ever a time when you couldn't concentrate?

Guidelines for Nursing Interventions

1. Use a firm and calm approach.
2. Use short, concise explanations or statements.
3. Remain neutral at all times.
4. Avoid power struggles.
5. Provide a consistent and structured environment.
6. Firmly redirect energy into appropriate and constructive channels.
7. Decrease environmental stimuli whenever possible.
8. Provide structured solitary activities. Tasks that require minimal concentration are best. Avoid groups and stimulating activities until client can tolerate that level of activity.

9. Provide frequent rest periods.
10. Provide high-calorie fluids and finger foods throughout the day.
11. Monitor client's sleep pattern, food intake, and elimination on a daily basis. (Constipation is often a problem.)
12. Teach client and family about the illness, and be sure both client and family have written information regarding client's medications.
13. Give client and family information about services in their community that can provide further information and support.

Psychopharmacology for Mania

Clients with a diagnosis of mania or bipolar disorder are often treated with lithium and other antimanic medications. Due to the nature of these drugs, it is especially important that client and family be informed of their effects. Tables 8 and 9 summarize the side effects and toxicity of these medications.

TABLE 8: SIDE AND TOXIC EFFECTS OF LITHIUM

Level	Signs*	Interventions
Expected Side Effects		
≤0.4–1.0 mEq/L (therapeutic levels)	Fine hand tremors, polyuria, mild thirst Mild nausea and general discomfort Weight gain	Symptoms may persist throughout therapy. Symptoms often subside during treatment. Change diet, exercise, nutritional management.
Early Signs of Toxicity		
<1.5 mEq/L	Nausea, vomiting, diarrhea, thirst, polyuria, slurred speech, muscle weakness	Withhold drug, draw blood lithium levels, reevaluate dose.
Advanced Signs of Toxicity		
1.5–2.0 mEq/L	Coarse hand tremor, persistent GI upset, mental confusion, muscle hyperirritability, EEG changes, incoordination	Use interventions outlined above or below, depending on severity.

(Continued on next page)

TABLE 8, CONTINUED

Level	Signs*	Interventions
Severe Toxicity		
2.0–2.5 mEq/L	Ataxia, serious EEG changes, blurred vision, clonic movements, large output of dilute urine, seizures, stupor, severe hypotension, coma. Death is usually secondary to pulmonary complications	There is no known antidote for lithium poisoning. Stop the drug and hasten excretion using gastric lavage and treatment with urea, mannitol, and aminophylline.
>2.5 mEq/L	Confusion, incontinence of urine or feces, coma, cardiac arrhythmia, peripheral circulatory collapse, abdominal pain, proteinurea, oliguria, and death	Hemodialysis may also be used in severe cases.

Data from Schere, J.C. (1995). *Nurses' drug manual* (pp. 631-632). Philadelphia: J.B. Lippincott; Lehne, R.A., et al. (1994). *Pharmacology for nursing care*, 2nd ed. (pp. 269-299). Philadelphia: W.B. Saunders.

*Careful monitoring is needed because the toxic levels of lithium are close to the therapeutic levels.

Client and Family Teaching: Lithium*

- Teach client and family that lithium treats the current problem *and* helps prevent relapse. It is therefore important to continue to take the drug after the current episode is resolved.
- Because therapeutic and toxic dosages are so close, lithium blood levels must be monitored closely.
- Assure client and family that lithium is not addictive.
- Encourage client to maintain a normal diet and normal salt and fluid intake (1500–3000 mL/day or six 12-oz. glasses). Explain that lithium decreases sodium reabsorption by the kidneys, which may cause sodium depletion. Low sodium intake causes a relative increase in lithium retention, which could lead to toxicity.
- Teach client to stop taking lithium if excessive diarrhea, vomiting, or diaphoresis occurs. Dehydration resulting from these can raise lithium levels to toxic amounts. *Instruct client to inform physician immediately if any of these problems occur.*

- Explain to client why client should not to take diuretics (water pills) while on lithium therapy.
- Teach client to take lithium with meals to avoid irritating stomach.
- Clients on long-term therapy should have renal and thyroid function monitored and should discuss follow-up with physician.
- Advise client to avoid taking over-the-counter medications without checking first with the physician.
- If weight gain is significant, refer client to physician or nutritionist.
- Inform client of local self-help and support groups that provide support for people with bipolar disorder and their families.
- Explain to client and family where to find more information.

*Data in this section from Maxmen, J.S., and Ward, N.G. (1995). *Psychotropic drugs: Fast facts*, 2nd ed. New York: W.W. Norton; Schatzberg, A.F., and Cole, J.O. (1991). *Manual of clinical psychopharmacology.* Washington, DC: American Psychiatric Press; Preston, J., and Johnson, J. (1995). *Clinical psychopharmacology made ridiculously simple.* Miami: Medmaster.

TABLE 9: OTHER ANTIMANIC MEDICATIONS

Drug	Type	Major Concerns/Side Effects
Carbamazepine (Tegretol)	Anticonvulsant	Agranulocytosis or aplastic anemia are most serious side effects.
		Blood levels should be monitored through first 8 weeks because drug induces liver enzymes that speed its own metabolism. Dose may need to be adjusted to maintain serum levels of 6–8 mg/L.
		Sedation is common problem; tolerance usually develops. Diplopia, incoordination, sedation signal excessive levels.
Valproic acid (Depakane)	Anticonvulsant	Baseline liver function tests should be performed and monitored at regular intervals. Hepatitis is rare but has been reported, with fatalities, in children.
		Signs and symptoms: fever, chills, right upper-quadrant pain, dark-colored urine, malaise, jaundice.
		Side effects: Tremors, GI upset, weight gain and alopecia.
Clonazepam (Klonopin)	Benzodiazepine	Same as those of all benzodiazepines (sedation, ataxia, incoordination).

PART II

PSYCHOTIC DISORDERS

SCHIZOPHRENIA

History

The following questions apply to the assessment of clients with symptoms of schizophrenia, including hallucinations, delusions, and paranoia.

- Does client have a personal or family history of schizophrenia?
- How old is client? (Schizophrenia usually first occurs during adolescence or early adulthood, although it can develop later.)
- Have all other medical and mental disorders, such as bipolar disorder, delirium, or ingestion or withdrawal from drugs, been ruled out as a cause of client's psychosis?

Assessing for Hallucinations

Hallucinations are *false sensory experiences* that have no basis in reality. The most common hallucinations in schizophrenia are auditory hallucinations.

Presenting Symptoms

- Client states that he or she hears voices.
- If client denies hearing voices, watch client's behavior for the following symptoms:
  - Eyes following something in motion that observer cannot see.
  - Staring at one place in the room.
  - Head turned to side as if listening.
  - Mumbling to self or conversing when no one else is present.
  - Inappropriate facial expressions, eyes blinking.
- If hallucinations are from other causes (drugs, alcohol, delirium), the underlying cause must be treated as soon as possible using accepted medical and nursing protocols.

Assessment Guidelines

- Assess for command hallucinations, such as voices telling the person to harm self or others.
- Determine when hallucinations seem to occur most often: in times of stress, at night, etc.

Sample Questions
- Have you ever seen or heard things that other people did not?
- Have you ever heard noises in your head that disturb you?
- Do the voices come from inside or outside your head?
  - Is it your voice or someone else's?
  - Does the voice speak your own thoughts?
- Is there more than one voice? Whose voices are they? Are they men's or women's voices? How old are they?
- When does this happen? What brings the voices on?
- How would you describe the voices? Are they friendly, arguing, hateful, controlling, terrorizing, constant?
- What do the voices say? Do they tell you to harm self or others?
- How do you usually cope with the voices?

Guidelines for Nursing Interventions
1. If voices tell client to harm self or others, take the necessary environmental precautions. If in hospital, use unit protocols. If in community, evaluate the need for hospitalization.
2. Communicate with client in direct, concrete, specific terms.
3. Decrease environmental stimuli (low noise, minimal activity).
4. Keep to simple, basic, reality-based topics of conversation.
5. Help client focus on one idea at a time.
6. Engage client in simple physical activities or tasks that channel energy (writing, drawing, craft projects).
7. Explore how client experiences the hallucinations.
8. Avoid using logic to convince client that he or she is wrong. Client will only become more defensive.
9. Be alert for signs of increasing fear, anxiety, or agitation.
10. Use words such as "your voices" or "the voices that you hear" when referring to the voices.
11. Accept the fact that the voices are real to the client, but you may state that you do not hear them. "I know that you hear your voices, but I do not hear any voices other than yours and mine."
12. Intervene with one-to-one, seclusion, or PRN medication (as ordered) when appropriate.

Assessing for Delusions

Delusions are *false, fixed ideas* that have no basis in reality.

Presenting Symptoms
- Client has fragmented, poorly organized, well organized, systematized, or extensive system of beliefs that are not supported by reality.
- The content of the delusions may be grandiose, persecutory, jealous, somatic, or based on guilt.

Assessment Guidelines
- Assess whether delusions have to do with someone trying to harm client and whether client is planning to retaliate against a person or organization. Assess whether precautions need to be taken.
- Determine when delusional thinking is the most prominent (when under stress, in presence of certain situations or people, etc.).

Sample Questions
- Did anyone try to use unusual means to force thoughts into your mind? To take some of your thoughts away? To stop or block your thoughts?
- Is your mind controlled by others?
- Are things on the TV or radio or in the newspapers especially meaningful to you? Do they contain special messages just for you?
- Do you think that someone or something is out to get you? Is anyone plotting against you?

Guidelines for Nursing Interventions
1. Assess for measures needed to protect client or others if client believes he or she needs to protect self against a specific person.
2. Be aware that clients' delusions represent the way they experience reality. If they believe someone is going to harm them, they are experiencing fear.
3. Do not argue with client's beliefs or try to correct them using facts. Doing so only makes client feel more defensive and isolated.

4. Try to convey an understanding of what client might be feeling: "If you believe that others are out to kill you . . . are you feeling frightened right now?"
5. Interact with clients on the basis of things in the environment. Try to distract clients from their delusions.
6. When possible, engage client in activities in which client can focus on reality-based phenomena.

Assessing for Paranoia

Paranoia is any *intense and strongly defended, irrational suspicion* that cannot be corrected by experiences or modified by facts or reality.

Presenting Symptoms
- Pervasive suspiciousness about everyone and their actions
- On guard, hyperalert, vigilant
- Blames others for consequences of own behavior
- Hostile, argumentative, and often uses threatening verbalizations or behavior
- Poor interpersonal relationships
- Delusions of influence, persecution, or grandiosity
- Often refuses medications because "nothing is wrong with me"
- May refuse food if client believes it may be poisoned

Assessment Guidelines
- Assess for suicidal or homicidal behaviors.
- Assess potential for violence.
- Assess need for hospitalization.

Sample Questions
- Do you believe that there is anything about you that has made other people jealous of you or prejudiced against you?
- Do you believe that you have special powers or unusual strengths?
- Do you believe you have ever received personal messages from God? From someone unusual?
- Do you think you are able to influence others or put thoughts into their minds?

- Do you believe that others are trying to hurt or kill you? Do others spy on you and wish you harm?
- Do you believe drugs or poisons have been put in your food or drink?

Guidelines for Nursing Interventions

1. Use nonjudgmental, respectful, and neutral approach with client.
2. Be honest and consistent with client regarding expectations and enforcing rules.
3. Use clear, simple language when communicating with client to minimize miscommunications.
4. Always keep your promises, and don't make promises that you cannot keep.
5. Explain to client what you are going to do before you do it to clarify your intentions.
6. Diffuse angry and hostile verbal attacks with a nondefensive stand.
7. Be aware of client's tendency to have ideas of reference. Do not do things in front of client that can be misinterpreted (laughing, whispering, or talking quietly when client can see but not hear what is being said).
8. Maintain a low level of stimuli and enhance a nonthreatening environment. Avoid groups.
9. Assess and observe client regularly for signs of increasing anxiety or hostility.
10. Provide verbal and physical limits when client's hostile behavior escalates. "We won't allow you to hurt anyone here. If you can't control yourself, we will help you."
11. Initially, provide solitary, noncompetitive activities that take some concentration. Later, introduce a game with one or more clients that takes concentration, such as chess or bridge.
12. If client is hospitalized, allow foods from home. Offer foods in cans (sardines, soups) or containers (yogurt, cottage cheese) or in their own skins (oranges, eggs, potatoes) to encourage client to maintain proper nutrition.
13. Encourage (do not push) client to discuss feelings (anxiety, fear). Refrain from dwelling on delusions.

Psychopharmacology in Schizophrenia

Tables 10 and 11 summarize the dosages, routes of administration, and characteristics of standard and atypical antipsychotic medications.

TABLE 10: STANDARD ANTIPSYCHOTIC MEDICATIONS

Drug	Routes	Acute (mg/day)*	Maintenance (mg/day)*	Special Considerations
Chlorpromazine (Thorazine)	PO, IM, R	200–1600	50–800	Increases sensitivity to sun. Highest sedation and hypotension effects; least potent.
Thioridazine (Mellaril)	PO	200–600	50–800	Known to cause retinitis pigmentosa in large doses; any diminished vision should be investigated. Low incidence of extrapyramidal side effects. High incidence of low blood pressure and cardiac effects.
Trifluoperazine (Stelazine)	PO, IM	10–60	2–80	Low sedation; good for withdrawn or paranoid symptoms. High incidence of extrapyramidal side effects. Neuroleptic malignant syndrome may occur.
Perphenazine (Trilafon)	PO, IM, IV	12–32	8–64	Helps control severe vomiting and intractable hiccups.
Mesoridazine (Serentil)	PO, IM	75–300	25–400	Among the most sedative; severe nausea/vomiting may occur in adults.
Fluphenazine (Prolixin)	PO, IM, SC	2.5–20	2–40	Among the least sedative.

Thioxanthenes

Drug	Routes	Acute (mg/day)*	Maintenance (mg/day)*	Special Considerations
Thiothixene (Navane)	PO, IM	6–30	6–60	High incidence of akathisia.

24

TABLE 10, CONTINUED

Drug	Routes	Acute (mg/day)*	Maintenance (mg/day)*	Special Considerations
Chloroprothixine (Taractan)	PO, IM	50–600	50–400	Weight gain common.
Butyrophenones				
Haloperidol (Haldol)	PO, IM	5–50	1–15	Low sedative properties; used in large doses for assaultive patients to avoid severe side effect of hypotension. Appropriate for the elderly; lessens chance of falls. High incidence of extrapyramidal side effects.
Dibenzoxapines				
Loxapine (Loxitane)	PO, IM	60–100	20–250	Possibly associated with weight reduction.
Dihydroindolones				
Molindone (Moban)	PO	50–100	15–225	Possibly associated with weight reduction.
Deconoate: Long-Acting				
Haloperidol deconoate (Haldol)	IM	0	50–100	Given deep muscle Z-track IM. Given every 4 weeks.
Fluphenazine decanoate (Prolixin)	IM	0	25	Given deep muscle Z-track IM. Effective 1–2 weeks.
Fluphenazine enanthate (Prolixin)	IM	0	25–75	Given deep muscle Z-track IM. Effective 3–4 weeks. Can cause acute dystonic reactions

Data from Kaplan, H.I., and Sadock, B.J. (1995). *Synopsis of psychiatry*, 6th ed. Baltimore: Williams & Wilkins; Maxmen, J.S., and Ward, N.G. (1995) *Psychotropic drugs: Fast facts*, 2nd ed. New York: W.W. Norton; Berkow, R., et al., eds. (1992). *Merck Manual*, 6th ed. Rahway, NJ: Merck Research Laboratories.

*Dosages vary with individual responses to antipsychotic agent used.

IM, intramuscular; PO, oral; R, rectal; SC, subcutaneous; IV, intravenous

TABLE 11: ATYPICAL ANTIPSYCHOTIC MEDICATIONS

Drug	Acute (mg/day)*	Maintenance (mg/day)*	Toxic/Side Effects	Special Considerations
Clozapine (Clozaril)	300–900	200–400 (start with low doses)	Agranulocytosis (0.8–2% of clients) Seizures Hypersalivation Persistent tachycardia	Used when clients fail to respond to other neuroleptics. Targets negative and positive symptoms. Weekly WBC required. High incidence of dose-related seizures. Can cause sedation, hypotension, tachycardia, and severe drooling.
Risperidone (Risperdal)		4–6	Insomnia (26%) Agitation (22%) EPS (17%) Headache (17%) Rhinitis (10%) Hypotension Anxiety (12%) Weight gain	Low EPS profile. Generally low side effects. Targets negative and positive symptoms. Start at 5 mg/day; gradually increase to minimize orthostatic hypotension. First-line antipsychotic.
Olanzapine (Zyprexa)	10–20	7.5–12.5–20	Agitation Insomnia (10.4%) Headache Nervousness (5.6%) Drowsiness Dizziness Akathisia (6.6%) Dry mouth (7.5%) Weight gain	Low side-effect profile, especially for cardiac and hematological problems. Targets negative and positive symptoms. First-line antipsychotic. Long half-life allows once-a-day dosage. Interactions with SSRIs and other antidepressants may occur.

TABLE 11, CONTINUED

Drug	Acute (mg/day)*	Maintenance (mg/day)*	Toxic/Side Effects	Special Considerations
Sertindole* (Serlect)		12–20–24	Rhinitis Decreases ejaculatory volume in men (17%); not associated with erectile disturbance or decreased libido Orthostatic hypotension Tachycardia	Can cause dose-related lengthening of QT interval on ECG. Monitor for signs of dizziness or lightheadedness due to ECG changes. Start with 4 mg/day and increase by 4 mg every 2–3 days to minimize orthostatic hypotension.

Data from Kaplan, H.I. and Sadock, B.M. (1995). *Synopsis of psychiatry*, 6th ed. Baltimore: Williams & Wilkins; Kane, J.M. (1995) Clinical psychopharmacology of schizophrenia. In G.O. Goddard, ed., *Treatment of psychiatric disorders*, 2nd ed., Vol. 1, pp. 970-986. Washington, DC: American Psychiatric Press; Littrel, K (1996). Olanzapine: An exciting new antipsychotic. *American Psychiatric Nurse's Association*, 8(4):4. Marder, S.R., Wirshing, W.C., and Ames, D. (1997) New antipsychotic drugs. In D.L. Dunner and J.F. Rosenbaum, eds., *Psychiatric Clinic of North America Annual of Drug Therapy*, pp. 195-207. Philadelphia: W.B. Saunders. American Psychiatric Association (1997). Practice Guidelines for the treatment of patients with schizophrenia. *American Journal of Psychiatry* (Suppl.) 154(4):21–23.

EPS, extrapyramidal side effects.

*Not yet FDA-approved as of this printing.

Client and Family Teaching: Schizophrenia

Medications

Client compliance tends to increase if client's family is supportive and involved, if client understands what to expect, and if client knows that the medication can be changed to decrease undesirable side effects.

- Explain what the medication can do for the client.
- Emphasize that medication needs to be taken regularly. Because schizophrenia is a relapsing disorder, it is extremely important to keep taking the drug, even though things may seem fine.
- Teach client and family what to do to lessen the severity of side effects that are not harmful to client.

- Explain that some side effects, although not harmful to client, may cause noncompliance because they are irritating. Examples include inner feelings of restlessness and nervousness or impotence. Tell client not to stop taking the drug for these reasons; most side effects can be treated. Instead, client should call *[give a name and number of person to be contacted for help]*.
- Teach client and family that if they observe toxic effects, they should discontinue the medication immediately, call *[give name and number]*, and take appropriate action until medical help is available.
- Direct client to avoid prolonged exposure to the sun and to wear sunscreen, sunglasses, long sleeves, and hats when in the sun.
- Advise client not to stop medication suddenly. Tolerance does not develop, but some clients report a rebound effect (nausea, vomiting, sleep disturbances) if drug is stopped suddenly.
- Assure client and family that the medications used to treat schizophrenia are not addictive.

Signs of Potential Relapse
When client or client's family recognize early warning signs, they can ward off potential relapse by seeking immediate medical attention. Both client and family need to be able to identify the warning symptoms that come before frank psychotic symptoms. These warning symptoms are unique to each client, but may include:

- Feeling of tension
- Difficulty concentrating
- Trouble sleeping
- Increased withdrawal
- Increased bizarre/magical thinking

Substances That Can Exacerbate a Psychotic Relapse
If client uses substances that can trigger a relapse, family support may influence client to minimize intake of these substances. The substances include marijuana, alcohol, and psychomotor stimulants such as amphetamines, cocaine, and crack cocaine.

PART III

ANXIETY DISORDERS

ANXIETY

Assessing for Anxiety

History
The following questions are intended as guidelines for obtaining a client's history when you assess for anxiety.

- Does client have a history of an anxiety disorder (phobia, obsessive compulsive disorder (OCD), post-traumatic stress disorder (PTSD), depersonalization disorder, panic attacks)?
- Does client have another psychological disorder (depression, substance abuse, sleep disorder, eating disorder)?
- Is client experiencing a loss or change (loss of job, move, death, retirement, illness, pregnancy)?
- Is anxiety secondary to other medical conditions (hyperthyroidism, multiple sclerosis)?

Presenting Symptoms
- Client reports feeling like he or she is going to die or has a sense of impending doom
- Narrowing of perceptions
- Difficulty concentrating, disorganization, inefficient problem solving
- Increase in vital signs (BP, P, R); sweat glands activated
- Pupils dilated
- Increased muscle tension
- Palpitations
- Urinary urgency/frequency
- Nausea
- Tightening of throat, unsteady voice
- Complaints of fatigue, difficulty sleeping
- Irritability

Assessment Guidelines

Tables 12 and 13 describe the perceptual field, ability to learn, and other characteristics of individuals who exhibit mild to moderate and severe to panic levels of anxiety.

TABLE 12: MILD TO MODERATE ANXIETY LEVELS

Mild	Moderate

Note: *Mild and moderate levels of anxiety can alert the person that something is wrong and can stimulate appropriate action.*

Perceptual Field

Perceptual field can be heightened	Perceptual field narrows. Person grasps less of what is going on.
Is alert and can see, hear, and grasp what is happening in the environment	Can attend to more *if pointed out by another* (selective attention).
Can identify things that are disturbing and are producing anxiety	

Ability to Learn

Able to work effectively toward a goal and examine alternatives	Able to solve problems, but not at optimal ability.
	Benefits from guidance of others.

Physical or Other Characteristics

Slight discomfort	Shakiness, voice tremors, change in voice pitch.
Attention-seeking behaviors	Difficulty concentrating.
Restlessness	Repetitive questioning.
Irritability or impatience	Increased muscle tension.
Mild tension-relieving behavior: foot or finger rapping, lip chewing, fidgeting	More extreme tension-relieving behavior: pacing, banging hands on table.
	Somatic complaints: urinary frequency and urgency, headache, backache, insomnia. Increased respiration and pulse rates.

TABLE 13: SEVERE TO PANIC ANXIETY LEVELS

Severe	Panic

Note: *In severe and panic levels of anxiety, the environment is blocked out. It is as if these events are not occurring. Severe and panic levels prevent problem solving and finding effective solutions. Unproductive relief behaviors are called into play, thus perpetuating a vicious cycle.*

Perceptual Field

Perceptual field is greatly reduced	Unable to focus on the environment.
Focus is on details or one specific detail; attention is scattered	Experiences the utmost state of terror and emotional paralysis. Feels he or she "ceases to exist."
Completely absorbed with self	In panic, hallucinations or delusions may take the place of reality.
May not be able to attend to events in the environment even when pointed out by others	

Ability to Learn

Unable to see connections between events or details	May be mute or have extreme psychomotor agitations leading to exhaustion.
Distorted perceptions	Disorganized or irrational reasoning.

Physical or Other Characteristics

Feelings of dread	Experience of terror.
Ineffective functioning	Immobility or severe hyperactivity or flight.
Confusion	Dilated pupils.
Purposeless activity	Unintelligible communication/inability to speak.
Sense of impending doom	
Somatic complaints: dizziness, nausea, headache, sleeplessness	Severe shakiness. Sleeplessness.
Hyperventilation	Out of touch with reality.
Tachycardia	Hallucinations or delusions likely.
Withdrawal	Severe withdrawal.
Loud, rapid speech	
Threats and demands	

Sample Questions

To obtain further information about a client's mental status, ask the client the following questions, adapting them to the current situation.

- Is there something you are very concerned about or afraid might happen?
- How does the future look to you?
- When you get frightened, what happens to you?
- Do you have times of great fear or anxiety attacks? What triggers them? How long do they last?
- Are there any distressing memories that keep coming back to you?
- Are there situations or places you avoid because they really upset you?

Guidelines for Nursing Interventions for Mild to Moderate Anxiety Levels

For mild to moderate levels of anxiety, the nursing goal is to reduce anxiety and prevent its escalation. The following guidelines provide a basis for working with patients whose anxiety levels do not exceed the moderate level.

1. Provide a safe, calm environment.
    a. Decrease environmental stimuli.
    b. Listen to client and offer reassurance that client can feel more in control.
2. Encourage client to talk about feelings and concerns.
3. Ask questions that clarify what client is saying.
4. Identify thoughts or feelings prior to the onset of anxiety. For example, you may ask, "What were you thinking right before you started to feel anxious?"
5. Identify what clients tell themselves to make themselves anxious.
6. Assess problem-solving skills and encourage client to engage in problem-solving activities.
7. Assess client's level of assertive communication skills and need for teaching.

8. Explore behaviors that have helped reduce anxiety in the past.
9. Provide outlets for working off excess energy (walking, dancing, exercising to music).
10. Teach relaxation techniques (deep-breathing exercises, meditation, progressive muscle relaxation.
11. Use role playing and rehearsal of stress-producing situations.
12. Refer client and family members to support groups, self-help programs, or advocacy groups when appropriate.

Guidelines for Nursing Interventions for Severe to Panic Anxiety Levels

In clients whose anxiety levels range from severe to panic, the primary goal is to provide safety measures and to reduce the client's anxiety.

1. Always remain with the person, or have a friend or relative remain with the person, when the person is experiencing a high level of anxiety.
2. Minimize environmental stimuli; move to a quiet setting.
3. Use a low-pitched voice, speak in simple statements, and repeat when necessary.
4. Reinforce reality if distortions occur.
5. Listen for themes in the conversation if thoughts are too disorganized.
6. Attend to physical needs (warmth, food, pain relief, need for family contact).
7. When safety is an issue, set physical limits as necessary.
8. Provide opportunities for client to pace or work off some tension when possible.
9. Assess client's need for medications or seclusion after other interventions have been tried.

Psychopharmacology for Anxiety Disorders

Table 14 identifies and describes medications that are commonly used to treat anxiety disorders.

TABLE 14: ANTIANXIETY MEDICATIONS

Generic Name (Trade Name)	Usual Daily Dose (mg/Day)	Action and Indication
Benzodiazepines (BZDs)		
Alprazolam (Xanax)	0.25–4.0	Increase GABA release and receptor binding at synapses. Show preferential effect on limbic system. Useful for short-term treatment of anxiety. Dependence and tolerance can develop.
Clonazepam (Klonopin)	0.5–20.0	
Diazepam (Valium)	4–30	
Lorazepam (Ativan)	2–6	
Oxazepam (Serax)	30–60	
Antihistamines		
Hydroxyzine hydrochloride (Atarax)	200–400	Depress subcortical centers. Produce no dependence, tolerance, or intoxication.
Hydroxyzine pamoate (Vistaril)	200–400	
Nonbenzodiazepines		
Buspirone hydrochloride (BuSpar)	15–80	Less sedating than benzodiazepines. Does not appear to produce physical or psychological dependence. Requires 3 weeks or more to be effective.
Beta Blockers		
Propranolol (Inderal)	30–80	Used to relieve physical symptoms of anxiety, as in stage fright. Acts by attaching to sensors that detect arousal messages.
Tricyclics		
Amitriptyline (Elavil)	150–300	Used to prevent panic attacks, phobias, and PTSD. Acts by regulating brain's reactions to serotonin. Clomipramine is helpful for some in lowering obsessions in OCD.
Clomipramine (Anafranil)	25–250	
Imipramine (Tofranil)	150–300	
Nortriptyline (Aventyl, Pamelor)	75–125	
Desipramine (Norpramin)	100–300	
MAOIs		
Phenelzine (Nardil)	45–90	Used to treat panic disorders, phobias, and PTSD. Acts by blocking reuptake of norepinephrine and serotonin in CNS.

(Continued on next page)

TABLE 14, Continued

Generic Name (Trade Name)	Usual Daily Dose (mg/Day)	Action and Indication
SSRIs		
Sertraline (Zoloft)	50–200	Used to treat OCD, panic,
Fluoxetine (Prozac)	10–40	agoraphobia, generalized anxiety
Paroxetine (Paxil)	20–50	disorder. Few anticholinergic
Fluvoxamine (Luvox)	100–300	effects.

OCD, obsessive-compulsive disorder; PTSD, post-traumatic stress disorder; MAOI, monoamine oxidase inhibitor; GABA, gamma-aminobutyric acid; SSRI, selective serotonin reuptake inhibitor.

Client and Family Teaching: Antianxiety Medications

- Instruct client and family not to increase the dose or frequency of ingestion without prior approval from the therapist. Benzodiazepines can be addictive.
- Explain that these medications reduce ability to handle mechanical equipment such as cars, saws, and other machinery.
- Caution client to avoid alcoholic beverages and taking other antianxiety drugs concurrently because the combination has the potential for dangerous central nervous system depression.
- Instruct client to avoid beverages that contain caffeine because it decreases the desired effects of the drug.
- Caution female clients to inform the physician immediately if pregnancy occurs. Benzodiazepines can increase the risk of congenital anomalies.
- Caution new mothers taking antianxiety medications not to breastfeed infants. Benzodiazepines are excreted in the milk and can have serious adverse effects on the infant.
- Caution client and family to avoid stopping benzodiazepines abruptly after three to four months of daily use; doing so may cause withdrawal symptoms. The drugs need to be tapered down.
- If client is elderly, explain to client and family that lower doses are often considered for elderly clients.

PART IV

CLINICAL BEHAVIORS REQUIRING INTERVENTION

SUICIDE

Assessing Potential for Suicide

History
The following questions are intended as guidelines for obtaining a client's history when you assess a client's potential for suicide.

- Does client have a history of suicidal attempts or self-mutilation?
- Is there a family history of suicide attempts or completion?
- Does client have a history of mood disorder, drug or alcohol abuse, or schizophrenia?
- Does client have a history of chronic pain, recent surgery, or chronic physical illness?
- Does client have a history of personality disorder (borderline, paranoid, antisocial)?

Presenting Symptoms

- Suicidal ideation—thoughts of harming self.
- Suicide attempt—attempt to kill self but failed this time.
- Deliberate self-harm syndrome—clients who mutilate their bodies.
- Hopelessness—degree of hopelessness is a crucial factor in suicide.

Assessment Guidelines

Tables 16 and 17 provide guidelines for assessing a client's risk for suicide. Table 16 is the SAD PERSONS scale, and Table 17 offers guidelines for assessing risk in children.

TABLE 15: SAD PERSONS SCALE

S	Sex	Men kill themselves three times more often than women, although women make attempts three times more often than men.
A	Age	High-risk groups: 19 years or younger; 45 years or older, especially the elderly of 65 years or over.
D	Depression	Studies report that 35–79% of those who attempt suicide manifested a depressive syndrome.
P	Previous attempts	Of those who commit suicide, 65–70% have made previous attempts.
E	ETOH	ETOH (alcohol) is associated with up to 65% of successful suicides. Estimates are that 15% of alcoholics commit suicide. Heavy drug use is considered to be in this group and is given the same weight as alcohol.
R	Rational thinking loss	People with functional or organic psychoses are more apt to commit suicide than those in the general population.
S	Social supports lacking	A suicidal person often lacks significant others (friends, relatives), meaningful employment, and religious supports. All three of these areas need to be assessed.
O	Organized plan	The presence of a specific plan for suicide (date, place, means) signifies a person at high risk.
N	No spouse	Repeated studies indicate that people who are widowed, separated, divorced, or single are at greater risk than those who are married.
S	Sickness	Chronic, debilitating, and severe illness is a risk factor.

Data from Patterson W., et al. (1983). Evaluation of suicidal patients: The SAD PERSONS scale. *Psychosomatics*, 24(4):343; Adam 1989; *Merck Manual* 1992; Mueller and Leon 1996.

TABLE 16: ASSESSING SUICIDAL RISK IN CHILDREN

Ask the child questions pertaining to the following areas:

1. **Suicidal fantasies or actions:**
   Ever had thoughts about, or the desire to, hurt or kill self?
   Ever made threats, or tried to, hurt or kill self?
2. **Concepts of what would happen:**
   What would happen if you tried to hurt or kill self?
   Do you think you would be injured, would die?
3. **Circumstances at the time of suicidal behavior:**
   What was happening at the time of the thought, the attempt?
   What was happening before the thoughts, the attempt?
   Was anyone with you at the time?
4. **Previous experience with suicidal behavior:**
   Have you ever thought of killing or tried to kill yourself before?
   Do you know anyone who thought about killing, tried to kill, or killed self?
   (Explore the child's perceptions of the event.)
5. **Motivation for suicidal behavior:**
   Why did you want to kill yourself; why did you try?
   Did you want to get even with someone, frighten someone?
   Did you want someone to rescue you?
   How are you feeling (hopeless, rejected, unloved, guilty)?
   Do you have frightening thoughts, hear voices saying kill self?
6. **Experience and concepts of death:**
   What happens when people die; where do they go?
   How often do you think or dream about dying?
   Did you know someone who died? (Explore the event.)
   When do you think you will die; what will happen?
7. **Depression and other effects:**
   Feelings of sadness, anger, guilt, rejection
   Description of behaviors—fighting, crying, lack of concentration, fatigue, changes in eating and sleeping patterns, problems with peers, withdrawn, isolated
8. **Family and environmental situations:**
   School performance, worries about school failure and parents' reaction
   Major changes—new home, school, siblings, stepparents
   Losses—death, divorce, separation from parents, separation of parents, illness
   Family history of marital conflicts, depression, or suicide

Adapted From: Pfeffer, C.R. (1986). *The Suicidal Child.* New York: The Guilford Press.

Sample Questions
- When was the first time you thought about hurting or killing yourself?
- Do you believe now that you want to die?
- Have you made any plans within the last month to hurt or kill yourself?
- When you have suicidal thoughts, how long do they last?
- Do you believe you have control over these thoughts?
- Has something specifically happened that brings (brought) on these thoughts, such as a loss, move, drugs, physical abuse, financial disaster?
- Have you planned how you might hurt yourself?
- Do you have the means to carry out your plan?

Guidelines for Nursing Interventions
1. Determine the appropriate level of suicide precautions for the client (physician or nurse) even in the emergency room.
2. *Follow unit protocols.* Suicide precautions depend on risk, but may include:
   a. Arms' length constraint (one-to-one with staff member at all times)
   b. One-to-one contact with staff at all times, but client may attend activities off the unit, maintaining one-to-one contact
   c. Knowing the client's location at all times on the unit and staff escort while client is off the unit
3. If there is fear of imminent harm, restraints may be required.
4. For high-risk clients, hospitalization may be necessary.
5. If a client is to be managed outside the hospital, alert client's family, lover, and/or friends to the risk and treatment plan and inform them of signs of deepening depression, such as a return or worsening of hopelessness.
6. If the client is to be managed on an outpatient basis, then consider the following steps (Slaby 1994):
   a. Rally social support.

b. Initiate appropriate psychopharmacotherapy, psychotherapy, or sociotherapy.
   c. Give client and client's family and friends the psychiatric clinician's telephone number, as well as that of a backup clinician or emergency room where they can go if the clinician is unavailable.
   d. Schedule a return visit (even the next day if it is felt that the decision not to hospitalize may need to be reconsidered).
   e. Alert friends and family to signs such as increasing withdrawal, preoccupation, silence, and remorse.
   f. Keep careful records in all instances documenting why a client was or was not hospitalized.
7. If the client is to be managed on an outpatient basis, give medication in a limited amount, e.g., a 5-day supply.
8. Form a written no-suicide contract with the client, such as "I will not kill myself for any reason, and if I should feel suicidal, I will (a) talk to a staff member, or (b) talk to my therapist."

VIOLENCE

Assessing Potential for Violence

History
Use the following questions as guidelines to assess a client's potential for violence.
- Does client have a history of violence?
- Does client have a history of paranoia?
- Does client ingest alcohol or drugs?
- Does client have a history of mania or agitated depression?
- Is a personality disorder present that might make client prone to rage, violence, or impulse dyscontrol?
- Does client have command auditory hallucinations?
- Does client have a cognitive disorder (dementia or delirium)?

Presenting Symptoms
- Violence is usually preceded by:
  - Hyperactivity, e.g. pacing. *This is the most important predictor of imminent violence.*
  - Increasing anxiety and tension: clenched jaw, fist, rigid posture, or fixed facial expression
  - Shortness of breath, sweating, and rapid pulse
  - Verbal abuse and profanity
- Recent acts of violence, including property violence
- Alcohol or drug intoxication
- Carrying a weapon or object that may be used as a weapon (e.g., fork, knife, rock)

Assessment Guidelines
- Does client have a violent wish or intention to harm another?
- Does client have a plan?
- Does client have the availability or means to carry out the plan?
- Consider demographics: sex (male), age (14–24), socioeconomic status (low support system).

Sample Questions
- Do you feel compelled or driven to do things you don't want to do?
- Have you ever been fired/evicted/arrested? If so, why did this happen?
- What do you do when you get very upset?
- Have you ever lost control of yourself? Ever thrown/broken things? Ever hit/attacked anyone?
- Do you get into more fights than other people in your neighborhood?

Guidelines for Nursing Interventions
1. *Always* minimize personal risks. Stay at least one arm's length away from client. Give client a lot of space.
2. Set limits at the onset.

Direct Approach
- "Violence is unacceptable."
- Describe the consequence (restraints, seclusion).
- Best for confused or psychotic clients.

Indirect Approach
- "You have a choice: you can take this medication and go into the interview room (or hallway) and talk, or you can sit in the seclusion room until you feel less anxious."
- Best for clients who are *not* confused or psychotic.

3. To reduce anxiety, either leave the door open in the interview room, or use a hallway if you feel uncertain of client's potential for violence. Other staff should be nearby.
4. Assess the need for chemical or physical restraints.
5. Empathetic verbal intervention is the most effective method of calming an agitated, fearful, panicky client: "It must be frightening to be here and to be feeling out of control."
6. Keep voice calm and speak in a low tone.
7. Call client by name, introduce yourself, and orient client as necessary.
8. Refrain from responding to profanity or verbal abuse by personalizing or defensive thoughts or behaviors. Verbal abuse is a defense against feelings of helplessness.
9. Encourage client to talk about angry feelings and wishes.
10. Keep environmental stimulation at a minimum. Lower lights; keep stereos down; ask clients and visitors to leave the area or have staff take client to another area.
11. When interpersonal and pharmacological interventions fail to control the angry client, physical interventions (restraints or seclusion) are the final resort. Alert hospital security and other staff in a quiet and unobtrusive manner before violent behavior escalates.
12. Carefully document client's behaviors, staff interventions, and client's responses before using seclusion/restraints.

Psychopharmacology for Chronic Aggression

Table 18 lists medications used to treat patients with chronic aggression related to various underlying illnesses or circumstances. Indications and relevant comments for each drug are also included.

TABLE 17: TREATMENT FOR CHRONIC AGGRESSION

Generic Group	Indications	Comments
Beta blockers, e.g., propranolol	Recurrent or chronic aggression in organically based violence: • Alzheimer's disease • Stroke • Huntington's disease Psychosis in which aggression is unrelated to psychotic thought	Often used in high doses (120–240 mg/day). Consistent and effective results may take 4–8 weeks.
Anticonvulsants	Bipolar disorder Borderline personality disorder Conduct disorder Episodic dyscontrol Post-traumatic stress disorder (PTSD) Central nervous system disorder	Carbamazepine—monitor bone marrow suppression and blood abnormalities. Valproic acid—monitor liver function and platelets.
Lithium	Mania-associated violence Uncontrolled rage triggered by nothing or minor stimuli (borderline personality disorder, PTSD)	Effective for violence in prisoners and mentally retarded clients. Does not affect aggressive behavior until therapeutic blood levels are reached.
Buspirone (BuSpar)	Cognitively impaired populations and possibly prison populations	Nonsedating and nonaddicting. Effectiveness takes 4–10 weeks to decrease aggression.

(Continued on next page)

TABLE 17, Continued

Generic Group	Indications	Comments
Nadolol	Diminishes assaultiveness in chronic paranoid schizophrenia	Few reports.
Trazodone	Aggression and agitation in demented and mentally retarded (does not impair cognition)	Do not use in males who cannot report priapism. Monitor for orthostatic hypotension.

Adapted from Maxmen, J.S., and Ward, N.G. (1995). *Psychotropic drugs: Fast facts,* 2nd ed., pp. 233-236. New York: W.W. Norton.

MANIPULATION

Assessing Presence of Manipulation

History
The following questions provide guidelines for assessing a client for presence of manipulation.

- Does client have a history of a personality disorder (borderline, antisocial, passive-aggressive)?
- Does client have a history of mania?
- Does client have a history of substance abuse?
- Does client have a history of unreliable or immature behaviors?

Presenting Symptoms
- Manipulation of staff, family, and others
- Playing one person against another (nurse against nurse, family member against staff, therapist against family member)
- Attempts to get special treatment or privileges
- Attention-seeking behaviors
- Use of somatic complaints to get out of doing things

- Lack of insight
- Denial of problems
- Focus on other people's problems (clients, staff, unit dynamics)

Assessment Guidelines
- Assess client for low frustration tolerance.
- Assess whether client resists limits set on negative behaviors.
- Note level of staff confusion and upset related to client pitting staff against staff.
- Assess whether client is seeking one staff member as "the one that really understands me" or "the nicest nurse," etc.
- Note whether client takes responsibility for his actions in family, staff, or unit altercations.

Sample Questions
- How do you feel when you don't get your way?
- What do you do when you don't get your way?
- Who do you trust?
- When do you feel the safest?
- In what situations do you feel the most vulnerable?

Guidelines for Nursing Interventions
1. State limits and the behavior you expect from the client in a matter-of-fact, nonthreatening tone.
2. Be sure the limits are:
   a. Appropriate, not punitive.
   b. Enforceable.
   c. Stated in a nonpersonal way. For example, "Alcohol is not allowed"; *not* "I don't want you to drink alcohol in the unit."
3. State the consequences if behaviors are not forthcoming. Written limits and consequences can be useful. Provide one copy for client and one for staff.
4. Be sure all staff understand the expectations, limits, and consequences discussed with the client to provide consistency. A written copy should be in Kardex or folder.

5. Follow through with the consequences.
6. Enforce all unit, hospital, group, and community center policies. State reasons for not bending the rules.
7. Be direct and confrontive if necessary in a neutral, factual manner, not out of anger.
8. Do *not:*
    a. Discuss yourself or other staff members with client.
    b. Promise to keep a secret for client.
    c. Accept gifts from client.
    d. Attempt to be liked, "the favorite," or popular with client.
9. Withdraw your attention when client's behavior is inappropriate.
10. Give attention and support when client's behavior is appropriate and positive.
11. Emphasize the client's feelings, not client's rationalizations or intellectualizations. Encourage client to express feelings.
12. Set limits on frequency and time of interactions with client, especially clients that involve therapists significant to client.
13. Encourage client to identify feelings or situations that trigger manipulative behaviors.
14. Role-play situations so that client may practice more direct and appropriate ways of relating.
15. Provide positive feedback when client interacts without use of manipulation.
16. When appropriate, see that client and family have names and numbers of appropriate community resources; e.g., Alanon, Alcoholics Anonymous, Parents Anonymous, Tough Love, etc.

APPENDICES

APPENDIX A

THE MINI-MENTAL STATE EXAMINATION*

ORIENTATION

5 ( ) What is the (year) (season) (date) (day) (month)?
5 ( ) Where are we (state) (county) (town) (hospital) (floor)?

REGISTRATION

3 ( ) Name three objects, and ask patient to repeat them (e.g., glass, window, table). One point for each correct. Continue until patient learns them.

ATTENTION AND CALCULATION

5 ( ) Serial 7s. One point for each correct response. Stop after 5 answers. (As an alternative, spell "WORLD" backwards.)

RECALL

3 ( ) Ask for three objects from registration section. One point for each correct.

LANGUAGE

2 ( ) Point to a pencil and a watch. Ask client to name each. One point for each correct.
1 ( ) Have client repeat: "No ifs, ands, or buts."
3 ( ) Have patient follow a three-stage command. "(1) Take paper in your right hand; (2) fold it in half; and (3) put it on the floor." One point for each correct.
1 ( ) Write the following in large letters: CLOSE YOUR EYES. Ask the patient to read and perform the task.
1 ( ) Ask client to write a sentence. Score one point if sentence has a subject, object, and verb.
1 ( ) Draw this design and have patient copy it.

TOTAL SCORE 30 Pts.___

Assess level of consciousness
Alert   Drowsy   Stupor   Coma

*Mini-Mental State Examination. Points are assigned for correct answers. Scores of 20 points or less indicate dementia, delirium, schizophrenia, or affective disorders alone or in combination. Such scores are not found in normal elderly people or in those with neuroses or personality disorders.

Adapted from Folstein, M.F., Folstein, S.E., McHugh, P.R. (1975). Mini-mental state: A practical method for grading the cognitive state of patients for the clinician. *Journal of Psychiatric Research*, 12:189–198.

APPENDIX B

RESOURCES AND REFERRAL INFORMATION

Note: The following is a list of clearinghouses that can help you locate support or self-help groups for clients. For a list of all self-help groups, go to **http://www.cmhc.com.selfhelp/** on the Internet.

Alabama	Birmingham area: 205-251-5912 (group information only)
Arizona	800-352-3792 (in Arizona); 602-231-0868
Arkansas	Northeast area: 501-932-5555 (group information only)
California	San Diego: 619-543-0412
	San Francisco: 415-772-4357
	Sacramento: 916-368-3100
	Modesto: 209-558-7454
	Davis: 916-756-8181
Connecticut	203-624-6982
Illinois*	312-368-9070; 312-481-8837
	Champaign area only: 217-352-0099
	Macon City: 217-429-HELP
Iowa	800-952-4777 (in Iowa); 515-576-5870
Kansas	800-445-0116 (in Kansas); 316-689-3843
Massachusetts	413-545-2313
Michigan*	800-777-5556 (in Michigan); 517-484-7373
Missouri	Kansas City: 816-822-7272
	St. Louis: 314-773-1399
Nebraska	402-476-9668
New Jersey	800-FOR-MASH (in New Jersey);
	201-625-9565
New York	New York City: 212-586-5770
	Westchester:** 914-949-0788, ext. 237
North Carolina	Mecklinberg area: 704-331-9500
North Dakota	Fargo area: 701-235-SEEK
Ohio	Dayton area: 513-225-3004
	Toledo area: 419-475-4449
Oregon	Portland area: 503-222-5555 (group information only)
Pennsylvania	Pittsburgh area: 412-261-5363
	Scranton area: 717-961-1234
South Carolina	Midlands area: 803-791-9227

Tennessee	Knoxville area: 423-584-9125
	Memphis area: 901-323-8485
Texas*	512-454-3706
Utah	Salt Lake City area: 801-978-3333 (group information only)
Virginia	Tidewater area: 757-340-9380

For international/national group contacts and/or directory:
American Self-Help Clearinghouse: 201-625-7101; TTY 625-9053; on the World Wide Web at **http://www.cmhc.com/selfhelp/**
National Self-Help Clearinghouse: 212-354-8525

OTHER INFORMATION HELPLINES IN THE UNITED STATES

O.D.P.H.P. National Health Information Clearinghouse	800-3365-4797 (in U.S.)
National Organization for Rare Disorders	800-999-NORD (in U.S.)
Alliance of Genetic Support Groups (genetic illnesses)	800-335-GENE (in U.S.)
National Empowerment Center (for mental health consumer/survivor groups)	800-POWER-2-U
National Mental Health Consumer's Self-Help Clearinghouse	800-553-4-KEY

SELF-HELP CLEARINGHOUSES IN CANADA

Calgary	403-262-1117
Nova Scotia	902-466-2011
Toronto*	416-487-4355
Prince Edward Island	902-628-1648
Vancouver	604-733-6186
Winnipeg	204-589-5599 or 633-5955

*Maintains listings of additional local clearinghouses operating within the state/province.
**Call Westchester for information on local clearinghouses in parts of upstate New York.

Adapted with permission from *Self-help sourcebook*, 6th ed., published by the American Self-Help Clearinghouse, Northwest Covenant Medical Center, Denville, NJ 07834-2995, 1997.

APPENDIX C

Selected Medications

The following pages contain in-depth information about drugs that are commonly used to treat clients with psychiatric mental health problems. This information has been standardized in a card-like format, and the drugs are arranged in alphabetical order for easier reference.

Benztropine Mesylate (Cogentin)
Buspirone Hydrochloride (BuSpar)
Carbamazepine (Tegretol, Epitol, Mazepine)
Chlorpromazine (Thorazine, Chlorazine)
Clozapine (Clozaril)
Diazepam (Valium)
Disulfiram (Antabuse)
Donepezil Hydrochloride (Aricept)
Fluoxetine Hydrochloride (Prozac)
Haloperidol (Haldol)
Imipramine Hydrochloride (Tofranil)
Lithium Carbonate/Citrate (Carbolith, Eskalith, Lithane, Lithizine, Lithonate, Lithobid)
Lorazepam (Ativan)
Olanzapine (Zyprexa)
Methylphenidate (Ritalin)
Nefazodone (Serzone)
Phenelzine Sulfate (Nardil)
Risperidone (Risperdal)
Sertraline Hydrochloride (Zoloft)
Tacrine (Cognex)
Zolpidem (Ambien)

BENZTROPINE MESYLATE
(Cogentin)

ANTIPARKINSONIAN

USES
1. Treatment of Parkinson's disease.
2. Treatment of extrapyramidal symptoms (except tardive dyskinesia) due to use of neuroleptic/antipsychotic medications.

ACTION
Cogentin is an anticholinergic agent that increases and prolongs the action of dopamine activity in the CNS, correcting neurotransmitter imbalances and minimizing involuntary movements.

DOSAGES & ROUTES

PO
Adult: 0.5–2 mg every day initially; gradually increase to 4–6 mg/day; for drug-induced extrapyramidal symptoms, 1–4 mg once or twice a day IM or PO.
Elderly: Use lower doses.

IM/IV
For acute dystonic reactions, 0.5–2 mg IM or IV.

CONTRAINDICATIONS
Acute narrow-angle glaucoma, pyloric or duodenal obstruction, peptic ulcers, prostatic hypertrophy, obstructions of the bladder neck, myasthenia gravis, children under three years of age. Rarely indicated for children.

CAUTIONS
The elderly and clients with cardiac, liver, or kidney disease or hypertension. Also clients taking barbiturates or alcohol.

SIDE EFFECTS
Autonomic: Dry mouth, nausea, restlessness; **CNS:** Sedation, vertigo, paresthesias; **Cardiovascular:** Palpitations, tachycardia; **GI:** Nausea, vomiting, constipation, paralytic ileus; **Genitourinary:** Dysuria, urinary retention; **Ocular:** Blurred vision, mydriasis, photophobia; **Other:** Anhidrosis (abnormal deficiency of sweat).

ADVERSE REACTIONS
CNS: CNS depression, mild agitation, muscle weakness, hallucinations, delirium, toxic psychosis, ataxia, numbness of the fingers.

REMARKS
The effects of benztropine are cumulative and may not be evident for 2–3 days. After 4–6 months of long-term maintenance antipsychotic therapy, can be used on an as-necessary basis or withdrawn. Some clients respond best to the medication given every day. Others do better with divided doses. Long-term use of benztropine with a neuroleptic can predispose client to tardive dyskinesia.

NURSING MEASURES
1. Monitor intake and output; observe for urinary retention.
2. Give medication after patient voids to reduce possibility of urinary retention.
3. Monitor for constipation; abdominal pain or distention indicate potential for paralytic ileus.
4. Indications of CNS toxicity (depression, excitement, hallucinations, etc.) warrant withholding drug. Inform physician immediately.

INFORM CLIENT
1. Avoid driving or operating equipment if drowsiness or dizziness occurs.
2. Tolerance to heat reduced due to reduced ability to sweat. Plan periods of rest in cool places.
3. Stop taking medication if CNS toxic effects, difficulty swallowing or speaking, or vomiting occurs. Inform physician immediately.
4. Monitor urinary output; watch for constipation.
5. Ask physician before using any medication, prescribed or OTC, while on benztropine.

BUSPIRONE HYDROCHLORIDE
(BuSpar)

ANTIANXIETY

USES
Management of anxiety disorders.

ACTION
The exact action of buspirone is not clear. It may exert a potent presynaptic dopamine antagonist effect in the CNS, resulting in increased dopamine at the synapses. It may also have an effect on serotonin receptors.

DOSAGES & ROUTES
PO Only

Adult and Elderly 5 mg 2–3 times daily; may increase 5 mg every 3–4 days; maintenance, 15–30 mg/day in 2–3 divided doses; not to exceed 60 mg/day.

CONTRAINDICATIONS
In clients with severe renal or hepatic impairment and clients on monoamine oxidase inhibitors (MAOIs).

CAUTIONS
Renal or hepatic impairment, pregnant/lactating women, elderly or debilitated clients.

SIDE EFFECTS
Dizziness, nausea, headache, nervousness, lightheadedness, and excitement, which generally are not major problems. Other, less common, problems include blurred vision, tachycardia, palpitations, paresthesia, abdominal distention.

ADVERSE REACTIONS
Overdose may produce severe nausea, vomiting, dizziness, drowsiness, abdominal distention, and/or excessive pupil constriction.

REMARKS
Advantages of BuSpar are that it is not sedating, does not produce a tolerance, and is not addicting. The drug has a more favorable side-effect profile than do the benzodiazepines.

NURSING MEASURES
1. Offer emotional support to anxious clients.
2. Liver and renal function tests and blood counts should be done regularly for clients on long-term therapy.
3. Assist with ambulation and put in place other safety features if dizziness and lightheadedness occur.

INFORM CLIENT AND FAMILY
1. Teach clients to inform their physicians:
   a. About any medications (prescription or nonprescription), alcohol, or drugs that they are taking.
   b. If they are now pregnant or plan to get pregnant.
   c. If they are breastfeeding an infant.
2. Do not drive a car or operate potentially dangerous machinery until client experiences the effects of this medication.
3. Notify physician of difficulty breathing, change in vision, sweating, flushing, cardiac problems.
4. Improvement may be noted in 7–10 days, but therapeutic effects may take 3–4 weeks or longer.

CARBAMAZEPINE
(Tegretol, Epitol, Mazepine)

ANTICONVULSANT, ANTINEURALGIC

USES
1. Management of generalized tonic-clonic seizures (grand mal) and psychomotor seizures.
2. Trigeminal neuralgia.
3. Potential mood stabilizer, particularly in acute mania. Used clinically, but not FDA-approved at present for this use.

ACTION
Reduces post-tetanic potentiation at synapses, preventing repetitive discharge.

DOSAGES & ROUTES: SEIZURES
PO Only (tablets, suspension,* and chewable tablets)

Adult   200 mg twice daily, gradually increase until response is attained; maintenance, 800–1200 mg/day.

Child (6–12)   100 mg twice daily, gradually increase until response is attained; maintenance, 400–800 mg/day.

*Oral suspensions produce higher peak concentrations. Going from tablets to suspension, give in smaller, more frequent doses.

CONTRAINDICATIONS
History of bone marrow depression; history of hypersensitivity to tricyclic antidepressants.

CAUTIONS
Impaired cardiac, hepatic, or renal function; pregnancy/lactation (crosses placenta, distributed in breast milk, accumulates in fetal tissue).

SIDE EFFECTS
Frequent: Drowsiness, dizziness, nausea and vomiting. **Infrequent:** Lethargy, visual abnormalities (spots before the eyes, difficulty focusing), dry mouth, headache, urinary frequency or retention, rash.

ADVERSE REACTIONS
Hematologic: Blood dyscrasias (aplastic anemia, agranulocytosis, thrombocytopenia, leukopenia, bone marrow depression). **Hepatic:** Abnormal hepatic function test results; jaundice; hepatitis. **Cardiovascular:** Congestive heart failure (CHF), edema, aggravation of coronary artery disease, arrhythmias, atrioventricular block, primary thrombophlebitis. Some complications have resulted in fatalities. **CNS:** Abrupt withdrawal may precipitate status epilepticus.

REMARKS
Monitoring drug levels has increased the safety of anticonvulsant therapy.

NURSING MEASURES
1. Monitor therapeutic serum level (3–12 μg/ml).
2. Assess for early toxic signs (fever, sore throat, mouth ulcerations, easy bruising, unusual bleeding, joint pain).
3. Observe frequently for recurrence of seizure activity.

INFORM CLIENT AND FAMILY
1. Blood tests should be repeated frequently during the first three months of therapy and at monthly intervals thereafter for 2–3 years.
2. Do not abruptly withdraw medications following long-term use (may precipitate seizures).
3. Avoid tasks that require alertness until response to drug is established.
4. Report visual abnormalities.

CHLORPROMAZINE
(Thorazine, Chlorazine)

ANTIPSYCHOTIC/NEUROLEPTIC — PHENOTHIAZINE

USES
1. Acute psychotic disorders (schizophrenia, manic phase of bipolar disorder); maintain remission of psychotic disorders.
2. Severe behavioral disturbances in children or clients with organic mental disorders.
3. Intractable hiccups, acute intermittent porphyria, tetanus, preoperatively, for nausea/vomiting.

ACTION
Blocks postsynaptic dopamine receptors in the cerebral cortex basal ganglia, hypothalamus, limbic system, brain stem, medulla. Therefore, it inhibits or alters dopamine release, thought to be related to suppression of clinical manifestations of schizophrenia. "Low potency" neuroleptic (EPS); high sedation and autonomic side effects.

DOSAGES & ROUTES: OUTPATIENT MAINTENANCE

	PO	IM	RECTAL SUPPOSITORY
Adult	Gradually increase over several days to maximum of 400 mg q4–6 hours.	25 mg—may give additional 25–50 mg in 1 hour if needed.	50–100 mg 3–4 times daily.
Child	0.55 mg/kg q4–6 hours.	None.	1.1 mg/kg every 6–8 hrs.
Elderly	(Debilitated) 25 mg tid.		

CONTRAINDICATIONS
Comatose states, alcohol or barbiturate withdrawal, bone marrow depression, pregnancy, lactation.

CAUTIONS
Seizure disorders, diabetes, hepatic disease, cardiac disease, glaucoma, prostatic hypertrophy, asthma.

SIDE EFFECTS
Autonomic: Dry mouth, nasal congestion, constipation/diarrhea, urinary retention/frequency, inhibition of ejaculation/impotence (men). **CNS:** EPS (pseudoparkinsonism, akathisia, dystonia); vertigo; insomnia. **Cardiovascular:** Orthostatic hypotension, hypertension, vertigo, EEG changes. **Endocrine:** Changes in libido, galactorrhea (women), gynecomastia (men). **Ocular:** Photophobia, blurred vision, aggravates glaucoma. **Other:** Weight gain, allergic reactions.

ADVERSE REACTIONS
CNS: Acute dystonias (painful neck spasms, torticollis, oculogyric crisis, convulsions); tardive dyskinesia (choreiform movements of tongue, face, mouth, jaw, extremities). Elderly and clients on drug for extended periods are more susceptible; condition is often irreversible. **Hematologic:** Agranulocytosis—stop drug immediately. **Neuroleptic malignant syndrome (NMS):** Life-threatening: rigidity, fever, low WBC, unstable BP, renal failure, tachycardia, tachypnea. *Hold all drugs.* Administer dantrolene sodium and bromocriptine immediately.

REMARKS
Food/antacids decrease absorption. Liquid preparation is absorbed more rapidly.

NURSING MEASURES
1. Check BP lying and standing (withhold if systolic is below 90) and notify physician.
2. Hold dose if EPS or jaundice.
3. Check frequently for urinary retention.
4. Check for constipation (avoid impaction).
5. Observe for fever, sore throat, and malaise; monitor CBC for blood dyscrasia.

INFORM CLIENT AND FAMILY
1. Rise slowly to sitting position and dangle legs 5 min. before standing to minimize hypotension.
2. Avoid sun. Use sunscreen when in direct light. Advise sunglasses for severe photosensitivity.
3. Avoid alcohol—enhances CNS depression.
4. Do not operate machinery if drowsiness occurs.

CLOZAPINE
(Clozaril)

ANTIPSYCHOTIC/NEUROLEPTIC — TRICYCLIC DIBENZODIAZEPINE DERIVATIVE

USES
Management of severely ill schizophrenic patients who fail to respond to other antipsychotic therapy.

ACTION
May involve antagonism of dopaminergic, serotoninergic, adrenergic, cholinergic neurotransmitter systems. Exact action unknown.

DOSAGES & ROUTES
PO Only

Adult Initially, 25 mg 1–2 times daily; may increase by 25–50 mg/day over 2 weeks to 300–450 mg/day; range, 200–600 mg/day; not to exceed 900 mg/day.

CONTRAINDICATIONS
Hypersensitivity to tricyclics, history of severe granulocytopenia; concurrent administration with other drugs having potential to suppress bone marrow function; clients who are CNS depressed or comatose or have myeloproliferative disorders.

CAUTIONS
Clients with a history of seizures; cardiovascular disease; impaired respiratory, hepatic, or renal function; alcohol withdrawal; urinary retention. Drug has potent anticholinergic effects, and extreme caution is advised for clients with prostatic enlargement or narrow-angle glaucoma. Also use with caution in pregnant or lactating women.

SIDE EFFECTS
Frequent: Sedation, salivation, tachycardia, dizziness, constipation. **Occasional:** Hypo- or hypertension, GI upset, nausea, vomiting, sweating, dry mouth, weight gain. **Rare:** Visual disturbances, diarrhea, rash, urinary abnormalities.

ADVERSE REACTIONS
Hematologic: Agranulocytosis; mild leukopenia. **CNS:** Seizures develop in about 5% of clients; up to 15% of clients on doses over 550 mg/day. Neuroleptic malignant syndrome (NMS) reported when clozapine is used concurrently with lithium/other CNS-active agents. **Other:** Dizziness/vertigo, drowsiness, restlessness, akinesia, agitation. **Cardiovascular:** Severe orthostatic hypotension (with or without syncope); marked tachycardia may occur in 25% of clients.

REMARKS
May take 2–4 weeks or as long as 3–6 months for therapeutic effects. Since 1–2% of people on clozapine develop agranulocytosis, weekly WBC counts must be done.

NURSING MEASURES
1. Check baseline WBC before initiating treatment.
2. Check weekly WBC count; hold drug if count falls below 3000 mm^3 and notify physician.
3. Check BP lying and standing to assess for potential orthostatic hypotension.
4. Observe for signs of agranulocytosis (sore throat, fever, malaise).
5. Make baseline assessment of behavior, appearance, emotional status, response to environment, speech pattern, and thought content.

INFORM CLIENT AND FAMILY
1. Know side effects and toxic effects of the drug and the need for a weekly WBC.
2. Avoid use of OTC drugs, alcohol, or CNS medications because of potential for severe drug interactions.
3. Report immediately the appearance of lethargy, weakness, fever, sore throat, malaise, mucous membrane ulceration, or other signs of possible infection.
4. Avoid operating machinery, driving, and other tasks that require alertness until response to the drug is established.
5. Inform physician if pregnancy occurs.
6. Do not breastfeed while taking Clozaril.

DIAZEPAM
(Valium)

ANXIOLYTIC (ANTIANXIETY AGENT) — BENZODIAZEPINE

USES
Anxiety disorders, short-term relief of anxiety symptoms; presurgical sedation to allay anxiety/tension; alcohol withdrawal; seizure disorders; anticonvulsant; skeletal muscle spasticity.

ACTION
Increases the action of gamma-aminobutyric acid (GABA). Benzodiazepines help GABA open a chloride channel in the postsynaptic membrane of many neurons, reducing neuron excitability.

DOSAGES & ROUTES

	PO	IM/IV
Adult	Anxiety: 2–10 mg 2–4 times daily.	2–10 mg 2–4 times daily.
	Muscle relaxant: 2–10 mg 2–4 times daily.	5–10 mg every 3–4 hours.
	Convulsions: 2–10 mg 2–4 times daily.	5–10 mg at 10-minute intervals.
	Alcohol withdrawal: 10 mg 3–4 times daily.	10 mg initially, then 5–10 mg every 3–4 hours.
Elderly	2.5 mg twice daily.	Convulsions: 2–5 mg (increase gradually as needed).

CONTRAINDICATIONS
Acute narrow-angle glaucoma, untreated open-angle glaucoma, during or 14 days after stopping MAOI therapy, depressed or psychotic clients without anxiety, first-trimester pregnancy, breastfeeding, shock, coma, acute alcohol intoxication.

CAUTIONS
Epilepsy, myasthenia gravis, impaired hepatic or renal function, drug abuse, addiction-prone clients. Injectable form used with extreme caution in the elderly, the very ill, and those with COPD.

SIDE EFFECTS
CNS: Sedation, vertigo, weakness, ataxia, decreased motor performance, confusion. **Ocular:** Double or blurred vision. **Skin:** Urticaria, rash, photosensitivity. **GI:** Weight change, dry mouth, constipation.

ADVERSE REACTIONS
CNS: This CNS depressant is fairly safe when used on its own, but used in combination with other CNS depressants, it can cause death. **Cardiovascular:** Tachycardia to cardiovascular collapse. **Metabolic:** Changes in liver or renal function tests. **Other:** Venous thrombosis or phlebitis at injection sites; rage reactions in some clients.

REMARKS
Diazepam can produce psychological and physical habituation, dependence, and withdrawal symptoms; it is recommended for short-term therapy (2–4 weeks). Use with caution in clients with histories of addiction. Withdrawal should be gradual to minimize withdrawal symptoms.

NURSING MEASURES
1. Obtain drug history of prescribed and over-the-counter medications.
2. Periodically monitor blood cell count and liver function test results during prolonged therapy.
3. Assess for unexplained bleeding, petechiae, fever, etc.
4. IM therapy: Aspirate back, administer deeply into large muscle mass; inject slowly; rotate injection sites.

INFORM CLIENT
1. Ask physician before taking alcohol or other CNS depressants while taking diazepam; can lead to respiratory depression.
2. Avoid driving or operating hazardous machinery if drowsiness or confusion occurs.
3. Avoid abrupt withdrawal of benzodiazepines.

DISULFIRAM
(Antabuse)

| ALCOHOL DETERRENT | ALDEHYDE DEHYDROGENASE INHIBITOR |

USES
Adjunct treatment for selected clients with chronic alcoholism who want to remain in a state of enforced sobriety. A form of aversion therapy.

ACTION
Inhibits hepatic enzymes from normal metabolic breakdown of alcohol, resulting in high levels of acetaldehyde, which causes the distressing symptoms of disulfiram-alcohol reaction.

DOSAGES & ROUTES
PO Only

Adult Initially, a maximum of 500 mg daily given as a single dose for 1–2 weeks; maintenance, 250 mg daily, not to exceed 500 mg daily.

CONTRAINDICATIONS
Severe heart disease, psychosis, hypersensitivity to disulfiram.

CAUTIONS
Diabetes, hypothyroidism, epilepsy, cerebral damage, nephritis, hepatic disease, pregnancy.

SIDE EFFECTS
Common side effects experienced during the first two weeks of therapy include mild drowsiness, fatigue, headache, metallic or garlic aftertaste, allergic dermatitis, and acne eruptions. Symptoms disappear spontaneously with continued therapy or reduced dosage.

ADVERSE REACTIONS
Disulfiram-alcohol reaction: Flushing or throbbing in head and neck, throbbing headache, nausea, copious vomiting, diaphoresis, dyspnea, hyperventilation, tachycardia, hypotension, marked uneasiness, vertigo, blurred vision, confusion. Can cause death.

REMARKS
Clients must abstain from alcohol intake for at least 12 hours before the initial dose of drug is administered.

NURSING MEASURES
1. Client must be able to demonstrate sobriety.
2. Client must be fully aware of drug's action when taken along with alcohol before treatment commences.
3. In severe disulfiram-alcohol reactions, supportive measures to restore BP and treatment for shock in a medical facility are vital.

INFORM CLIENT AND FAMILY
1. Avoid any substances that contain alcohol.
   a. **Ingestion:** Elixirs, cough syrups, vinegars, vitamin/mineral tonics; be aware that some sauces, soups, ciders, flavor extracts (vanilla, cherry) and some desserts (flaming, some cakes/pies) are made with alcohol.
   b. **Topical:** Mouthwash, body lotions, liniments, shaving lotion.
   c. **Inhalation:** Avoid inhaling fumes from substances that may contain alcohol, such as paints, wood stains, varnishes, and "stripping" compounds.
2. Carry a card stating that if client is found disoriented or unconscious, client may be having a disulfiram-alcohol reaction and telling the finder who to contact for medical care.
3. A disulfiram-alcohol reaction can occur within five to 10 minutes after ingestion of alcohol and can last 30–60 minutes or longer.
4. Reaction may occur with alcohol up to 14 days after ingesting disulfiram.

DONEPEZIL HYDROCHLORIDE
(Aricept)

CHOLINESTERASE INHIBITOR

USES
Treatment of mild to moderate dementia of the Alzheimer's type.

ACTION
The cholinergic system deteriorates in Alzheimer's disease. Donepezil inhibits the breakdown of endogenously released acetylcholine.

DOSAGES & ROUTES
PO
Adults and Elderly   Start with 5 mg daily dose. After 6 weeks, may raise to 10 mg daily.

CONTRAINDICATIONS
Hypersensitivity to donepezil or piperidine derivatives.

CAUTIONS
Cholinesterase inhibitors may increase gastric acid secretion. Therefore, clients should be monitored for gastrointestinal bleeding (especially those at increased risk of developing ulcers—history of ulcer disease, receiving nonsteroidal anti-inflammatory drugs.) Use with caution in clients who have a history of seizures. Prescribe with care to clients with asthma or obstructive pulmonary disease.

SIDE EFFECTS
Nausea, vomiting, diarrhea, insomnia, muscle cramps, fatigue, and anorexia.

ADVERSE REACTIONS
Syncopal episodes have been reported in association with the use of this drug.

NURSING MEASURES
1. Obtain an accurate list of other drugs client is taking. Use with anticholinergic drugs may interfere with the activity of anticholinergic medications.
2. Discuss with family and friends to determine who is to administer the medication to client to prevent incorrect dosages.

INFORM CLIENT AND FAMILY
1. Take the drug in the evening prior to retiring.
2. Drug may be taken with food.
3. If overdose is accidentally ingested, call a Poison Control Center to determine the latest recommendations for the management of an overdose of any drug.

FLUOXETINE HYDROCHLORIDE
(Prozac)

ANTIDEPRESSANT

USES
1. Prozac is an atypical antidepressant medication that is chemically unrelated to tricyclic antidepressants or monoamine oxidase inhibitors.
2. Has been found effective in clients with bulimia and obsessive-compulsive disorders.

ACTION
Fluoxetine is a potent serotonin reuptake blocker whose use results in an increase in the amount of active serotonin within the synaptic cleft and at the serotonin receptor site. Increased serotonin in these areas appears to modify affective and behavioral disorders.

DOSAGES & ROUTES
PO

Adult	20 mg/day; may reach 40–60 mg in divided doses; do not exceed 80 mg/day.
Elderly	Same as for adults.
Child	No dosage for children as yet established.

CONTRAINDICATIONS
Not to be taken within 14 days of an MAOI. Also, client must wait 5 weeks if going from fluoxetine to an MAOI.

CAUTIONS
Use with clients with concomitant systemic illness has not been studied extensively. Caution should be used with pregnant/lactating women, children, and the elderly. Caution should also be used with clients with liver disease or renal impairment and with clients who have had a recent myocardial infarction (MI).

SIDE EFFECTS
The most common side effects reported with fluoxetine hydrochloride are nausea, nervousness and anxiety, insomnia, and vertigo. When these side effects are severe, the drug is discontinued. If a rash or urticaria or both develop, the drug should be discontinued. Anorexia may appear in some people.

ADVERSE REACTIONS
See side effects.

REMARKS
Fluoxetine, like the tricyclic antidepressants and MAOIs, takes 2–5 weeks to produce an elevation of mood. Advantages of this drug are that there are fewer anticholinergic side effects and that there is a low incidence of cardiovascular effects. However, fluoxetine may impair judgment, thinking, and motor skills.

NURSING MEASURES
1. Fluoxetine hydrochloride is given in the early morning without consideration of meals.
2. Assess clients who are potentially suicidal for suicidal thoughts or actions. Carefully observe taking of medication.
3. If client is underweight and experiences anorexia, alert the physician to evaluate continuation of medication.

INFORM CLIENT
1. If rash or urticaria appears, notify physician immediately.
2. Do not drive or operate hazardous machinery if drowsiness occurs.
3. Avoid alcoholic beverages.

HALOPERIDOL
(Haldol)

ANTIPSYCHOTIC/NEUROLEPTIC — BUTYROPHENONE

USES
Psychotic disorders; helps control remissions in schizophrenia; children with combative, explosive hyperexcitability *(use is controversial)*; control of tic and vocal utterances of Gilles de la Tourette's disorder; acute mania and acute and chronic organic psychosis; drug-induced psychosis (LSD).

ACTION
Blocks binding of dopamine to the postsynaptic dopamine receptors in the brain.

DOSAGES & ROUTES

PO
- Adult: 0.5–2.0 mg 2–3 times daily.
- Elderly: Elderly or debilitated clients may require smaller doses than adults.
- Child: Not for children under 3; for children 3–12 years, 0.15 mg/kg/day in 2–3 divided doses.

IM
(Severe) 3–5 mg every 1–8 hours to control symptoms, then give PO.

CONTRAINDICATIONS
Hypersensitivity, Parkinson's disease, depression, seizures, coma, alcoholism, lithium therapy.

CAUTIONS
Elderly; anticoagulants; glaucoma, prostatic hypertrophy, urinary retention, asthma, pregnancy/lactation.

SIDE EFFECTS
Autonomic: Dry mouth, nasal congestion, constipation/diarrhea, urinary retention/frequency, inhibition of ejaculation and impotence (men). **CNS:** EPS. **Cardiovascular:** Orthostatic hypotension, hypertension, dizziness, EEG changes. **Endocrine:** Libido changes, galactorrhea (women), gynecomastia (men). **Ocular:** Photophobia, blurred vision, aggravation of glaucoma. **Other:** Weight gain, allergic reactions.

ADVERSE REACTIONS
CNS: Acute dystonias (painful neck spasms, torticollis, oculogyric crisis, convulsions); tardive dyskinesia (choreiform movements of tongue, face, mouth, jaw, extremities; often irreversible. The elderly and those on drug for extended periods are more susceptible; neuroleptic malignant syndrome (NMS) may occur within 24–72 hours (fever, rigidity, renal failure, arrhythmias, etc.) Hold drug and give dantrolene sodium or bromocriptine immediately. **Hematologic:** Agranulocytosis—stop drug immediately. **Hepatic:** Jaundice; clinical picture resembles hepatitis.

REMARKS
"High potency" neuroleptic; higher incidence of EPS; lower incidence of sedation and orthostatic hypotension. Effect of Haldol deconoate E or D given IM using Z track may last 1–3 weeks.

NURSING MEASURES
1. Check for signs of tardive dyskinesia (protrusion of tongue, puffing cheeks, chewing or puckering mouth) and report to physician immediately.
2. Observe for other signs of EPS and jaundice.
3. Check for orthostatic hypotension (take BP lying and standing). Withhold if systolic is 80 or below.
4. Check frequently for urinary retention.
5. Check for constipation (avoid impaction).
6. Observe for fever, sore throat, and malaise, and monitor CBC for indications of a blood dyscrasia.
7. Monitor renal function during long-term therapy.
8. Monitor blood levels every week.

INFORM CLIENT
1. Rise slowly to a sitting position and dangle legs 5 min. before standing to minimize hypotension.
2. Use sunscreen when in direct light.
3. Avoid alcohol—it enhances CNS depression.
4. Do not operate machinery if drowsiness occurs.

IMIPRAMINE HYDROCHLORIDE
(Tofranil)

ANTIDEPRESSANT — TRICYCLIC

USES
Depression (major, bipolar, or dysthymia); organic affective disorders and obsessive-compulsive disorders; adjunctive treatment in childhood enuresis and in bulimia; agoraphobia with panic attacks and generalized anxiety disorder.

ACTION
TCAs block the reuptake of norepinephrine and serotonin into their presynaptic neurons.

DOSAGES & ROUTES

	PO	IM
Adult	50 mg/day to start in 1–4 divided doses up to 200 mg/day for outpatients.	Do not exceed 100 mg/day in divided doses.
Elderly	Used with caution—usually start at lower dose. Geriatric clients start on 30–40 mg daily.	
Child	Childhood enuresis: 25 mg before bedtime. Depression (children >12 years): 30–40 mg/day initially.	

CONTRAINDICATIONS
MI, cardiac disease, renal or hepatic impairment. Death may occur if used with MAOI; may be cautiously used with MAOI in refractory depression. May cause fatal cardiac arrhythmias in clients with hyperthyroidism. Use with caution in children, adolescents, elderly, especially those with cardiac, respiratory, cardiovascular, hepatic, or GI diseases.

CAUTIONS
Renal or hepatic disease, narrow-angle glaucoma. Assess potential for suicide. Monitor clients with seizure disorders; TCAs lower seizure threshold.

SIDE EFFECTS
Anticholinergic: Dry mouth/nasal passages, constipation, urinary hesitancy, esophageal reflux, blurred vision. **Cardiovascular:** Orthostatic hypotension, hypertension, palpitations. **CNS:** Tachycardia, vertigo, tinnitus, paresthesia. **Endocrine:** Galactorrhea, libido change, ejaculation and erectile disturbances, delayed orgasm. **Other:** Weight gain, cholestatic jaundice, fatigue.

ADVERSE REACTIONS
Autonomic: Intracardiac conduction slowing. **Cardiovascular:** MI, CHF, arrhythmias, heart block, cardiotoxicity, CVA, shock. **CNS:** Ataxia, neuropathy, EPS. **Hematologic:** Bone marrow depression, agranulocytosis. **Psychiatric:** Hallucinations, hypomania, mania, exacerbation of psychosis.

REMARKS
Before receiving TCAs, clients need a thorough physical and cardiac workup.

NURSING MEASURES
1. Monitor BP (lying and standing) every 2–6 hours when initiating therapy.
2. Observe suicidal clients closely during initial therapy.
3. Supervise ingestion to prevent hoarding of drug.
4. Assess for urinary retention.
5. Monitor liver function and CBC (assess for signs of cholestatic jaundice and agranulocytosis).
6. Dispense only small amount of drug if client is to be discharged.
7. Monitor diabetic clients closely, especially during early therapy; hypo- or hyperglycemia may occur.
8. Observe for hypomania, mania, and seizure activity.

INFORM CLIENT
1. Rise slowly to prevent hypotensive effects.
2. Do not drive or use hazardous machinery if drowsiness or vertigo occurs.
3. Ask physician before taking OTC drugs.
4. Discuss use of alcohol with physician before taking this drug.
5. Mood elevation may take 1–4 weeks.

LITHIUM CARBONATE/CITRATE
(Carbolith, Eskalith, Lithane, Lithizine, Lithonate, Lithobid)

ANTIMANIC — LITHIUM

USES
Primarily used to control, prevent, or diminish manic episodes in people with bipolar depression (manic-depressive psychosis). Also used experimentally in alcoholism, premenstrual syndrome, drug abuse, phobias, eating disorders, and rage reactions in selected patients.

ACTION
Lithium is an alkali metal salt that behaves much like sodium; lowers norepinephrine and serotonin concentrations by inhibiting release and enhancing reuptake by neurons. Therapeutic, side, and toxic effects of lithium may be related to partial replacement of sodium by lithium in membrane action.

DOSAGES & ROUTES
PO

Adult   Acute mania, 600 mg tid; maintenance dose, 300 mg tid or qid.
Elderly   Reduce to 600–900 mg/day to produce low serum concentration of about 0.5 mEq/L.
Child   Not labeled for pediatric use.

CONTRAINDICATIONS
Pregnancy/lactation, significant cardiovascular or renal disease, schizophrenia, severe debilitation, dehydration, sodium depletion.

CAUTIONS
The elderly, thyroid disease, epilepsy, concomitant use with haloperidol or other antipsychotics, parkinsonism, severe infection, urinary retention, diabetes.

SIDE EFFECTS
Below 1.5 mEq/L: Hypothyroidism and impairment of kidney's ability to concentrate urine. Polyuria, polydipsia, lethargy, fatigue, muscle weakness, headache, mild nausea, fine hand tremor, inability to concentrate; ankle edema. Symptoms disappear during continued therapy.

ADVERSE AND TOXIC EFFECTS
1.5–2.0 mEq/L: Vomiting, diarrhea, muscle weakness, ataxia, dizziness, slurred speech, confusion.
2.0–2.5 mEq/L: Blurred vision, muscle twitching, severe hypotension, persistent nausea and vomiting. Thyroid toxicity is common. **2.5–3.0 mEq/L or more:** Urinary and fecal incontinence, seizures, cardiac arrhythmias, peripheral vascular collapse, death.

REMARKS
Monitor serum lithium levels during drug therapy. Therapeutic range is very narrow, and potential for toxic effects is high. During acute stage, blood levels rise to 1.00–1.4 mEq/L. Maintenance therapy blood levels: 0.8–1.2 mEq/L. Side/toxic effects common at higher doses (1.5 mEq/L or more). Before client starts lithium, measure BUN, T4, T3, and TSH levels and do an ECG.

NURSING MEASURES
1. If serum lithium levels are above 1.5 mEq/L or if client has persistent diarrhea, vomiting, excessive sweating, infection, or fever, check with physician before giving dose.
2. Check urine specific gravity periodically; teach client to do so at home (normal: 1.005–1.025).
3. Administer lithium with meals.
4. Ensure that client is well hydrated.

INFORM CLIENT
1. Drink plenty of liquids (2–3 L/day) during initial therapy and 1–1.5 L/day during remaining therapy.
2. Know side and toxic effects of lithium and call physician immediately if problems arise.
3. Have blood lithium levels measured at intervals as directed to regulate dosage/prevent toxicity.
4. Regular diet with average salt intake (6–8 g) to keep serum lithium level in therapeutic range.
5. Avoid alcohol.
6. Antibiotics and nonsteroidal antiinflammatory agents can increase lithium levels.
7. Caffeine can lower lithium levels.

LORAZEPAM
(Ativan)

ANTIANXIETY AGENT — BENZODIAZEPINE

USES
1. Treatment of anxiety disorders associated with depression.
2. Preoperative sedation.
3. Nausea and vomiting associated with chemotherapy in cancer.

ACTION
CNS depressant, especially limbic system and reticular formation. Enhances action of inhibitory neurotransmitter gamma-aminobutyric acid (GABA), producing a calming effect. Can suppress spread of seizure activity and can directly depress motor nerve and muscle function, creating some muscle relaxation.

DOSAGES & ROUTES
PO

Adult	For anxiety	2–3 mg daily in 2–3 divided doses.
	For insomnia	2–4 mg at bedtime.
Elderly	For anxiety	0.5–1 mg/day; may increase gradually.
	For insomnia	0.5–1 mg at bedtime.

CONTRAINDICATIONS
Acute narrow-angle glaucoma, alcohol intoxication, pregnancy/lactation, children under 12.

CAUTIONS
Renal or hepatic dysfunctions, elderly or debilitated clients, clients with history of drug abuse/addictions; clients on other CNS depressants (narcotics, barbiturates, alcohol) may have a synergistic effect increasing CNS depression. May reduce digoxin excretion, increasing potential for toxicity.

SIDE EFFECTS
Frequent: Drowsiness, fatigue, dizziness, incoordination. **Occasional:** Blurred vision, slurred speech, hypotension, headache. **Rare:** Paradoxical CNS restlessness, excitement in elderly or debilitated clients.

ADVERSE REACTIONS
Can have pronounced withdrawal symptoms (seizures, pronounced restlessness, insomnia, abdominal/muscle cramps) with abrupt withdrawal from the drug.

REMARKS
When used preoperatively, lorazepam is usually given IM or IV. Monitor BP (lying and standing) for orthostatic hypertension; if systolic drops 20 mmHg or more, stop medication and notify physician. Monitor respiration frequently if drug is given IV.

NURSING MEASURES
1. Assess for history of glaucoma, substance use, allergies, past reactions to benzodiazepines.
2. Obtain current list of medications.
3. If client is on long-term therapy, assess CBC and liver function (with physician).
4. Ascertain that client has written information about medications that covers side effects, doses, precautions, and other information.

INFORM CLIENT AND FAMILY
1. Avoid tasks that require alertness or motor skills (driving, operating machinery).
2. Ask physician before taking over-the-counter medications.
3. Do not drink alcohol or take other CNS depressants while taking this medication.
4. Do not stop medication abruptly.

OLANZAPINE
(Zyprexa)

ATYPICAL ANTIPSYCHOTIC

USES
1. First-line treatment for schizophrenia; targets both positive and negative symptoms of schizophrenia.
2. Other psychotic illnesses.

ACTION
Olanzapine blocks various serotonin (5-HT2A) receptors and dopamine (D2) receptors. It also antagonizes dopamine D1–D4 receptors, serotonin 5-HT2C and 5HT3 receptors, and the alpha 1-adrenergic and H1 histaminic receptors.

DOSAGES & ROUTES
PO

Adult   Given in 5 mg to 10 mg doses once daily (at bedtime), with target of 10 mg/day; 15 mg does not seem to be more effective than 10 mg/day. Range of 5–20 mg/day.

CONTRAINDICATIONS
Clients with known hypersensitivity to olanzapine.

CAUTIONS
Olanzapine seems to have a good side-effect profile and low potential interactions. Carbamazepine may increase olanzapine clearance by 50% at a dose of 200 mg bid; nicotine may increase olanzapine clearance by 40% in smokers.

SIDE EFFECTS
Frequent: Psychomotor slowing (somnolence, asthenia) and psychomotor activation (agitation, nervousness, insomnia, hostility) and dizziness, weight gain. **Infrequent:** At higher doses, anticholinergic effects (constipation, dry mouth, increased appetite).

ADVERSE REACTIONS
None known.

REMARKS
Mild transient dose-related increases in hepatic transaminase and prolactin levels may occur; these increases resolve spontaneously and do not require discontinuation of the drug.

NURSING MEASURES
1. Assess client and family for knowledge about schizophrenia.
2. With physician's cooperation, get baseline hepatic profile.

INFORM CLIENT AND FAMILY
1. Have client and family report any concerns about the drug.
2. Give information about community support groups.
3. Give dose at bedtime.
4. Do not drive or operate machinery.
5. Use stool softeners if client becomes constipated.

METHYLPHENIDATE
(Ritalin)

CNS STIMULANT

USES
1. Attention-deficit disorder (children 6 years of age or older).
2. Narcolepsy.
3. Occasionally, depression in the elderly.

ACTION
Releases catecholamines directly into synaptic clefts and thus onto postsynaptic receptor sites. Blocks reuptake of catecholamines, prolonging their actions. Also serve as false neurotransmitters.

DOSAGES & ROUTES
PO

Adult	Doses may start at 5 mg 2–3 times/day; dose range for adults is 10 mg/day to not more than 60 mg/day; usual is 20–40 mg/day.
Elderly	Depression: usually maintained on 2.5–20 mg/day.
Child	6 years or older: usual starting dose is 5 mg tid (breakfast and lunch); most are maintained on 60 mg/day, and should be monitored by prescribing physician.

CONTRAINDICATIONS
Glaucoma, hypertension, heart problems, or history of Tourette's syndrome. People with seizure disorders may experience increase in the number, duration, and/or severity of seizures.

CAUTIONS
Can cause growth delay in children. May interact with other substances and medications, such as alcohol, antidepressants (MAOIs and TCAs), OTC medications, health food products containing Ma Huang. Serious problems may also develop if clients take any other amphetamine-type or diet drugs.

SIDE EFFECTS
Frequent: Most common are nervousness and sleeplessness. Other reactions include loss of appetite, weight loss, nausea, dizziness, heart palpitations, increase in blood pressure, stomach upset, and growth delay in children with prolonged therapy. **Occasional:** Dizziness, dysphoria, joint pain, fever.

ADVERSE REACTIONS
Can cause an increase in seizures in people with seizure disorders, chest pain, dysrhythmias. Can have serious interactions with other medications and over-the-counter preparations.

NURSING MEASURES
Obtain complete list of health food products and medications client is taking, prescribed and OTC. Check with pharmacy if not certain if Ritalin is compatible with client medications.

INFORM CLIENT AND FAMILY
1. Ask parents to discuss "Drug Holidays" with prescriber to help avoid side effect of growth delay.
2. Drug may have serious side effects when mixed with other substances. Have client or family check with physician before taking over-the-counter medications, other drugs, or health food products from other sources.
3. Take Ritalin shortly before meals, not after 12 noon or 1 PM (children) or 6 PM (adults); stimulant effect may keep people awake.
4. If child must take Ritalin during school hours, ask pharmacist to provide additional empty, labeled container. Place no more than one week's medication in the bottle. Be sure the medication is secured with school official.
5. Once client dosage is stabilized, Ritalin can be given in an extended-release form. Client should swallow these tablets whole; never crush or chew.
6. Keep tablets dry, tightly capped, away from direct heat.
7. Keep out of reach of children and pets.

NEFAZODONE
(Serzone)

ANTIDEPRESSANT — SSNRI

USES
Treatment of depression

ACTION
Nefazodone and one of its active metabolites exert dual effects on serotonergic neurotransmission by blocking serotonin type 2 (5HT2) receptors and inhibiting serotonin uptake. The parent compound (NEF) and another active metabolite also exhibit affinity for the 5-HT1c receptor. Nefazodone lacks anticholinergic or antihistaminic effects, but exhibits some affinity for alpha 1-adrenergic receptors.

DOSAGES & ROUTES
PO

Adult	Start on 100–200 mg/day (50–100 mg bid), maintenance dose from 300–500 mg/day (150–250 mg bid)
Elderly	Start on 50–100 mg/day (25–50 mg bid), maintenance dose from 150–250 mg/day (75–175 mg bid)

CONTRAINDICATIONS
To avoid potentially life-threatening cardiotoxicity, clients on nefazodone should not take nonsedating antihistamines (terfenadine [Seldane], astemizole [Hismanal]). Drugs such as alprazolam (Xanax) and triazolam (Halcion) require dosage reductions when used concomitantly. Nefazodone should not be used with MAOIs or within 14 days of terminating MAOIs. Contraindicated in clients with known hypersensitivity to nefazodone and components of the formulation or other phenyl-piperazine antidepressants.

CAUTIONS
This drug should be used only if clearly needed by pregnant/lactating clients. Lactating women should not breastfeed while receiving nefazodone. Use with caution with pre-existing hypotension or labile circulation, pre-existing liver disease, renal disease, heart disease, or a history of seizures or allergies. Suicide assessment is needed, and prescriptions should be written for smallest quantity of tablets consistent with good client management.

SIDE EFFECTS
Frequent: Sleepiness, dry mouth, nausea, dizziness (especially when standing), constipation, confusion, incoordination, blurred vision or changes in vision. **Infrequent:** Irregular heartbeat, skin rash.

ADVERSE REACTIONS
Cardiovascular: Sinus bradycardia and first-degree A–V block. **Genitourinary:** Nefazodone is structurally related to trazodone, which has been associated with the occurrence of priapism. There have been no reported cases; however, if a client presents with a prolonged or inappropriate erection, he should discontinue therapy and consult the physician immediately.

NURSING MEASURES
1. Give the drug bid in divided doses.
2. Observe suicidal clients for suicidal actions if hospitalized; give the smallest number of tablets consistent with good management if in the community.
3. Teach measures for combating orthostatic hypotension in case the client experiences dizziness upon rising.

INFORM CLIENT
1. Do not drive or operate machinery if drowsiness occurs.
2. Drug may take 2–3 weeks before therapeutic effects are noted.
3. Warn of excessive sedation during initial therapy.

PHENELZINE SULFATE
(Nardil)

ANTIDEPRESSANT   MAOI

USES
1. Depression that is refractory to tricyclic antidepressant therapy, especially atypical depression; agoraphobia, and hypo-chondriasis; panic disorders.

ACTION
Effect is thought to be due to irreversible inhibition of MAO, increasing the concentration of epinephrine, norepinephrine, serotonin, and dopamine in the presynaptic neurons and at the receptor site.

DOSAGES & ROUTES
PO
Adult   15 mg tid; increase rapidly to 60 mg/day until therapeutic level is noted.
Elderly   Prone to side effects; if >60 years of age, MAOIs may be contraindicated.
Child   Not used with children.

CONTRAINDICATIONS
Confused or noncompliant client (due to hypertensive crisis, CVA, or hyperpyrexia states that can lead to death due to untoward interactions with certain foods and cold remedies); CHF, cardiovascular or cerebrovascular disease, impaired renal function, glaucoma, history of severe headaches, liver disease; elderly or debilitated clients; pregnant clients; paranoid schizophrenia.

CAUTIONS
Depression accompanying alcoholism or drug addiction, manic-depressive states, suicidal tendencies, agitated clients, and people with chronic brain syndromes, or a history of angina pectoris.

SIDE EFFECTS
Constipation, dry mouth, vertigo, orthostatic hypotension, drowsiness or insomnia, weakness, fatigue, weight gain, hypomania, mania, blurred vision, skin rash. Muscle twitching is common.

ADVERSE REACTIONS
Hypertensive crisis: Intense occipital headache, palpitation, stiff neck, fever, chest pain, bradycardia or tachycardia, intracranial bleeding. **Hepatic:** Jaundice, malaise, right upper-quadrant pain, change in color or consistency of stools.

REMARKS
Because of severe interactions with some foods and medications, clients need comprehensive teaching, teaching aids, and supervision. **High-tyramine foods:** beer, red wine, aged cheese, dry sausage, fava beans, brewer's yeast, smoked fish, liver, avocados, bologna. May use chocolate and coffee in moderation. **Drugs:** meperidine (Demerol), epinephrine, local anesthetics, decongestants, cough medications, diet pills; most OTC drugs.

NURSING MEASURES
1. Monitor BP for orthostatic hypotension every 2–4 hours during initial therapy.
2. Assess for potential signs of hypertensive crisis.
3. Observe for marked changes in mood (hypomania, mania).
4. Monitor intake/output and frequency of stools.
5. Have client dangle legs 5 min. before standing.
6. Depressed clients are at risk for suicide; monitor for potential suicidal behaviors.

INFORM CLIENT AND FAMILY
1. Inform client and family clearly and carefully about foods and medications to avoid. REVIEW IN DETAIL.
2. Instruct clients taking MAOIs to wear a medical identification tag or bracelet.
3. Ask physician before taking OTC drugs.
4. Avoid all alcohol.
5. Go to emergency room immediately if signs and symptoms of hypertensive crisis are suspected. Phentolamine (Regitine) can be given for hypertensive crises.

RISPERIDONE
(Risperdal)

ATYPICAL ANTIPSYCHOTIC

USES
Potent antipsychotic agent; targets negative (withdrawal, apathy, negativism) as well as positive (hallucinations, delusions, paranoia, hostility) symptoms of schizophrenia.

ACTION
A potent antagonist at 5HT2a and D2 receptors (serotonin and dopamine).

DOSAGES & ROUTES
PO

Adult — Dose range 4–16 mg/day (6 mg/day dose most effective for many).
Elderly — Dose range 1–4 mg/day.

CONTRAINDICATIONS
Clients known to be hypersensitive to Risperidone.

CAUTIONS
Can cause orthostatic hypotension and tachycardia. Because of these reactions, it should be started at low doses (0.5 mg in the elderly and 1.0 mg for adults). Risperidone is associated with dose-related EPS, although often minimal in therapeutic range. Use with caution in clients with a history of seizures.

SIDE EFFECTS
Frequent: Sedation, insomnia, rhinitis, coughing, back or chest pain, erectile problems in men, weight gain, decreased sexual interest. Initial dosing especially may cause orthostatic hypotension and tachycardia or syncope. In some clients, causes anorexia, polyuria, polydipsia and/or an increase in dream activity. **Occasional:** Extrapyramidal side effects (EPS) and increases in plasma prolactin can lead to galactorrhea and menstrual disturbances in some women.

ADVERSE REACTIONS
A number of cases of neuroleptic malignant syndrome (NMS) and rare cases of priapism have been reported.

NURSING MEASURES
1. Teach client what the medication can and cannot do. This drug can target some of the negative symptoms, and that should be included in client teaching.
2. Give client a list of the possible side effects and those reactions that warrant contacting the prescribing provider: palpitations, erectile or sexual disinterest problems that might threaten compliance, or dizziness.
3. Teach client to sit on bed 5 minutes when getting out of bed in the morning to avoid dizziness when getting up and potential falls.
4. Check to see if client has a history of seizures.

INFORM CLIENT AND FAMILY
1. When starting on medication, be careful driving cars, working around machinery, and crossing streets. Medication can make people sleepy and perhaps dizzy, especially initially.
2. Do not suddenly stop taking medication even if there is no immediate return of symptoms. Relapse is a very high risk in the weeks and months after medications have been stopped.
3. Instruct client or family member to notify the physician if client has sore throat during the first several months of treatment, if NMS appears (client should have a fact sheet on NMS), or if client is going to have general or dental surgery or is experiencing chest pain or tachycardia or palpitations.

SERTRALINE HYDROCHLORIDE
(Zoloft)

ANTIDEPRESSANT — SSRI

USES
1. Major depression.
2. Obsessive-compulsive disorder (OCD)

ACTION
Enhances serotonergic activity in the CNS by blocking the reuptake of serotonin by neuronal presynaptic membranes. Has only a very weak effect on dopamine and norepinephrine reuptake.

DOSAGES & ROUTES
PO

Adult   Initially, 50 mg/day once daily with morning or evening meal; may be increased no sooner than every week up to a maximum of 200 mg/day.

Elderly   Initially, 25 mg/day once daily as above. May increase by 25 mg q2–3 days.

CONTRAINDICATIONS
Use within 14 days of MAOIs; hypersensitivity to the drug. Safety of this drug with children and in pregnancy has not been established.

CAUTIONS
Severe hepatic or renal insufficiency, elderly and debilitated clients, suicidal clients, and clients with a history of seizures or mania.
Drug interactions: Cimetidine can increase sertraline concentrations; diazepam concentrations may be increased; decrease in tolbutamide may occur; and may increase bleeding in clients on Warfarin.

SIDE EFFECTS
Frequent: Dizziness, headache, tremor, insomnia, somnolence, fatigue, agitation, nausea, dry mouth, loose stools or constipation, sexual dysfunction. **Occasional:** Increased sweating, dyspepsia, anorexia, nervousness, rhinitis, abnormal vision. **Rare:** Rash, vomiting, frequent urination, palpitations, paresthesia, twitching.

NURSING MEASURES
1. Zoloft is best given in the morning.
2. If hospitalized, watch for signs of "cheeking" of medications (that is, not swallowing medications, but rather holding them under the tongue or in the cheek for the purpose of saving them and taking an overdose at a later time.
3. If client is extremely depressed, client should be given only one-week supply at a time.

INFORM CLIENT AND FAMILY
1. Improvement may take 1–3 weeks, although it is often noticed after a much shorter period of time.
2. Caution client against prematurely discontinuing the therapy, which can result in a relapse. In general, medication should continue for at least 6 months to a year after symptoms have subsided.
3. Have client and family assess for signs of improvement in symptoms, especially in areas such as depressed mood and loss of interest or pleasure in usual activities.
4. Have client and family watch for signs of suicidal ideation.

TACRINE
(Cognex)

REVERSIBLE CHOLINESTERASE INHIBITOR

USES
Can help in mild to moderate dementia in people with Alzheimer's disease. Appears to reverse 6 months of dementia's progress.

ACTION
Cholinergic system deteriorates in Alzheimer's dementia. Tacrine inhibits breakdown of endogenously released acetylcholine.

DOSAGES & ROUTES
PO

Adult 40 mg/day, with more improvement noticed at 80–160 mg/day. Because of 2-hour half-life, needs qid dosing.

Start at 10 mg qid (40 mg) and continue 6 weeks if tolerated. Every 6 weeks, increase dose by 10 mg qid. If tolerated, go to 160 mg/day (40 mg qid).

CONTRAINDICATIONS
Can be hepatotoxic in some clients.

CAUTIONS
Because of elevation in liver enzymes, clients need frequent liver function testing. Other drugs can raise or lower tacrine levels. Anticholinergic agents can reverse tacrine's effects. Cholinergic agents risk increased toxicity with tacrine. Smoking can also lower tacrine levels.

SIDE EFFECTS
Flu-like symptoms without fever, gastrointestinal (nausea, diarrhea, dyspepsia, anorexia, vomiting).

ADVERSE REACTIONS
Elevation of transaminase (ALT/SGPT).

REMARKS
Because of possibility of transaminase elevation, liver functions should be done and ALT levels should be monitored weekly for 6 weeks after each dose increase. This is the most common reason for dropouts.

NURSING MEASURES
Smoking and certain medications can alter tacrine levels. Ascertain whether client smokes, and be sure that client has informed prescribing physician/nurse of all medications client is taking. Check for effects on tacrine levels.

INFORM CLIENT AND FAMILY
1. Serum transaminase level must be monitored monthly.
2. Remind family to let physician know of any and all medications that client is taking, since tacrine levels can easily be altered by some medications.
3. This drug is not a panacea, but it may be very useful in the early stages of dementia.

ZOLPIDEM
(Ambien)

NONBENZODIAZEPINE SEDATIVE/HYPNOTIC

USES
Short-term treatment of insomnia.

ACTION
Zolpidem is thought to bind to the GABA receptors in the CNS, giving the drug sedative, anticonvulsant, and antianxiety properties.

DOSAGES & ROUTES
PO

Adult	10 mg immediately before bedtime.
Elderly	5 mg immediately before bedtime.

CONTRAINDICATIONS
Safety has not been established for pregnancy, lactation, and children under the age of 18.

CAUTION
People with renal or hepatic dysfunction. Clients with history of drug abuse/addictions; depressed or suicidal clients; elderly or debilitated clients.

SIDE EFFECTS
Frequent: Drowsiness, vertigo, double vision, headache, drugged feeling, euphoria, insomnia, and nausea. **Occasional:** Palpitations, myalgia, sinusitis, rash.

ADVERSE REACTIONS
Rarely, doses over 10 mg have been associated with psychotic reactions and anterograde amnesia.

NURSING MEASURES
1. Establish baseline history of sleep pattern.
2. Assess for other medications that can cause CNS depression that the client may be taking, including level of alcohol use.
3. Identify other methods client has used previously to induce sleep.
4. Assess for adverse reactions and side effects.

INFORM CLIENT AND FAMILY
1. Zolpidem is only for short-term use. Explore other methods of inducing sleep.
2. Do not drive or use machinery once drug has been taken.
3. Take immediately before sleep.
4. Do not take other medications or OTC medications while taking this drug unless approved by physician.
5. Do not consume alcohol while taking this drug.

APPENDIX C, continued

Selected Medications—Year 2000 Update

Buprenorphine (Buprenex)
Fluvoxamine Maleate (Luvox)
Gabapentin (Neurontin)
Lamotrigine (Lamictal)
Quetiapine (Seroquel)

BUPRENORPHINE
(Buprenex)

PARTIAL U-OPIOID RECEPTOR AGONIST

USES
1. Relief of moderate to severe pain.
2. Being studied as a adjunct treatment in opioid addiction.

ACTION
Binds with opioid receptors within the CNS, thereby altering pain perception and emotional response to pain.

DOSAGES & ROUTES
USA-Injectable only-0.3 mg/ml (IM or IV)
Europe-Sublingually

Adults, Children Over 13:	0.3 mg q6h as needed: may repeat 30–60 min after initial dose. May increase to 0.6 mg and/or reduce dosing interval to q4h if necessary.
Children 2–12:	2-6 mcg/kg q4–6h.
Elderly:	Usual dose 0.15 mg q6h prn.

CONTRAINDICATIONS
None significant.

CAUTIONS
1. Impaired hepatic/renal function, elderly debilitated, head injury, respiratory disease, hypertension, hypothyroidism, Addison's disease, acute alcoholism, urethral stricture.
2. Pregnancy: Crosses placenta. Prolonged use during pregnancy may produce withdrawal symptoms in neonate.
3. Lactation: Breast-feeding not recommended.

DRUG INTERACTIONS
CNS depressants; MAO inhibitors may increase CNS or respiratory depression, hypotension. May decrease effects of other opioid analgesics.

ALTERED LAB VALUES
May increase amylase lipase.

SIDE EFFECTS
Frequent: Sedation, dizziness. **Occasional:** Headaches, hypotension, nausea/vomiting, hypoventilation, sweating. **Infrequent**: Dry mouth, pallor, visual abnormalities, injection site reaction.

ADVERSE REACTIONS
Overdose: Cold and clammy skin, weakness, confusion, severe respiratory depression, pinpoint pupils, extreme somnolence progressing to convulsions, stupor, coma.

NURSING MEASURES
1. If respirations 12/min or lower (20/min in children) withhold medication and contact physician.
2. Assess onset, type, location, and duration of pain.
3. Monitor for change in respiration, BP, rate/quality of pulse.
4. Initiate deep breathing, coughing exercises, particularly in those with impaired pulmonary function.
5. Change client's position q2–q4 h.
6. Record effects of medication; e.g., onset of relief of pain.

INFORM CLIENT AND FAMILY
1. Teach client:
   a. Not to exceed prescribed dose
   b. Avoid alcohol or benzodiazepines
   c. Avoid tasks that require alertness, motor skills (e.g., driving a car).
   d. Change position frequently to avoid dizziness.

FLUVOXAMINE MALEATE
(Luvox)

ANTIDEPRESSANT

USES
Treatment of obsessive-compulsive disorders (OCD). Treatment of depression.

ACTION
Selectively inhibits serotonin neuronal uptake in CNS, producing an antidepressant effect.

DOSAGES & ROUTES

Adult	50 mg at bedtime, increased by 50 mg q 4–7 days to a maximum of 300 mg a day. Doses over 100 mg in 2 divided doses.
Children (8-17)	25 mg at bedtime, increased by 25 mg q 4–7 days up to a maximum of 200 mg a day.

CONTRAINDICATIONS
Do not take within 14 days of an MAO inhibitor, concurrent astemizole or Terfenadine therapy.

CAUTION
Use with caution if a client has a history of seizures, heart disease, kidney disease, liver disease, or allergies. This drug should be used only if clearly needed during pregnancy. This medication appears in breast milk.

REMARKS
This drug may interact with a variety of other medications both prescribed and over-the-counter. For example, lithium, all antidepressants (SSRIs and others), dexfenflurramine, warfarin, phenytoin, benzodiazepines, cabamazepine, clozapine, methadone, propranolol, any MAO inhibitors, haloperidol, and others. A careful drug history is warranted for anyone going on this medication.

SIDE EFFECTS
Frequent: Nausea, vomiting, constipation, upset stomach, delayed ejaculation, decreased libido, urinary frequency, drowsiness, headache, anxiety, tremors, trouble sleeping, dry mouth.
Infrequent: Dizziness, fatigue, constipation, rash, pruritis, back pain, visual disturbances.

ADVERSE REACTIONS
Cardiac: Rapid, pounding, or irregular heartbeat, chest pain. **CNS**: Confusion, disorientation, unusual uncontrolled movements especially around face. **Hematological**: Bruising or bleeding. **General**: Flu-like symptoms (fever, chills).

NURSING MEASURES
1. For clients on long-term therapy, baseline liver/renal function test and baseline blood counts need to be done and repeated periodically throughout treatment.
2. Perform a suicide assessment and evaluate risk factors. Does client's history include past suicidal behavior or threats? Identify client's support system.
3. Obtain a drug history from client as to over-the-counter, prescription (especially psychoactive medications, cardiac, and many others) and recreational drugs client currently uses. How much and how often does client use alcohol? Be sure there is good documentation in client's chart, and prescribing health care worker is well informed.

INFORM CLIENT AND FAMILY
1. Drug may take up to 4 weeks before improvement is noted.
2. Helpful interventions for common side effects include:
    a. Sunglasses for photosensitivity.
    b. Sugarless gum and sips of water for dry mouth.
    c. Rise and move slowly to avoid hypotensive effects.
    d. Avoid tasks requiring motor skills (driving a car) until response to drug is established.
3. Because of drug interactions client should avoid alcohol.

GABAPENTIN
(Neurontin)

ANTICONVULSANT

USES
Gabapentin is indicated as adjunctive therapy in the treatment of partial seizures with and without secondary generalization in adults with epilepsy. Neuropathic pain.

ACTION
May be related increased gamma-aminobutyric acid (GABA) synthesis rate, increased GABA accumulation, or binding to as-yet undefined receptor sites in the brain to produce anticonvulsant activity. Exact mechanism is not known.

DOSAGE & ROUTES
PO-Capsules (100 mg, 300 mg, 400 mg)

Adult	Effective dose is 900–1800 mg given in divided dose (TID). Titration to an effective dose can take place rapidly giving 300 mg on day 1 (HS), 300 BID (Q12h) on day 2, and 300 mg TID on day 3 (q8h) and continue dose up to 1800 mg when indicated.
Elderly	In elderly clients with compromised renal function, doses need to be adjusted.

CONTRAINDICATIONS
Gabapentin is contraindicated in clients who have demonstrated hyperactivity to the drug or its ingredients.

CAUTION
Use with caution in clients with renal impairment. Dose needs to be modified. Use with caution in pregnant women. Safety and effectiveness has not been has not been established in children under 12.

SIDE EFFECTS
Frequent: Fatigue, somnolence, dizziness, ataxia, nystagmus, tremor, diplopia, rhinitis, hypertension. **Infrequent:** Weight gain, dyspepsia, myalgia, nervousness, dysarthria, pharyngitis, diplopia, nausea, and vomiting.

ADVERSE REACTIONS
Difficulty breathing or tightening of the throat, swelling of lips or tongue, rash, slurred speech, drowsiness, diarrhea.

NURSING MEASURES
1. Review history of seizure disorder (type, onset, intensity, frequency, duration, level of consciousness).
2. Assess for seizure activity. Provide safety measures as needed.
3. Obtain baseline assessment, including vital signs.
4. Obtain information on all other medications (prescription, nonprescription, nutritional supplements or herbal products) that client is taking.
5. Obtain history of alcohol frequency and amount, and other recreational drugs that may affect the way the medication will work.

INFORM CLIENT AND FAMILY
1. Drug should not be abruptly discontinued because of the possibility of increasing seizure activity.
2. Drug should be taken as prescribed.
3. Gabapentin may cause dizziness, somnolence, and other symptoms of CNS depression; therefore, clients should be advised to refrain from driving a car or operating complex machinery.
4. Teach client to tell physician if they:
    a. Are about to become pregnant
    b. Are breast feeding

LAMOTRIGINE
(Lamictal)

ANTICONVULSANT (ANTIEPILEPTIC DRUG OF THE PHENYLTRIAZINE CLASS)

USES
1. Adjunctive treatment of partial seizures in adults with epilepsy.
2. Used experimentally in the treatment of refractory bipolar depression.

ACTION
The precise mechanism by which lamotrigine exerts its anticonvulsant action are unknown. It is thought to be related to the drug's effect on sodium channels.

DOSAGES & ROUTES
PO Tablets (25 mg, 100 mg, 150 mg, 200 mg)

Adults, Elderly, Children Over 16:	(If receiving enzyme-inducing antiepileptic drugs (AEDs), but valproate. Recommend as add-on therapy) 50 mg once/day for 2 weeks, followed by 100 mg/day in 2 divided doses for 2 weeks. *Maintenance Dose:* Dose may be increased by 100 mg/day every week up to 300–500mg in 2 divided doses.
Adults, Elderly, Children Over 16:	(If receiving combination therapy of valproic acid and enzyme-inducing antiepileptic drugs (AEDs): 25 mg every other day for 2 weeks followed by 25 mg once/day for 2 weeks. *Maintenance Dose:* Dose may be increased by 25–50 mg/day every 1–2 weeks up to 150 mg/day in 2 divided doses.
Children 16 Or Under:	**NOT** approved for children under 16 years of age. See Adverse TOXIC reactions.

CONTRAINDICATIONS
Children under 16 years of age. The incidence of severe, potentially life-threatening rash in pediatric clients is very much higher than that reported in adults using Lamotrigine (1in 50 to 1 in 100 pediatric clients.)

CAUTIONS
1. Use with caution in clients with:
   a. Renal impairment
   b. Hepatic function impairment
   c. Cardiac function impairment
2. Pregnancy: Can reduce fetal weight, delay ossification noted in animals.
3. Lactation: Breast-feeding not recommended. Pregnancy Category C.

SIDE EFFECTS
Frequent: Dizziness, double vision, headache, ataxia (muscular in-coordination), nausea, blurred vision, somnolence, and rhinitis. **Occasional:** Pharyngitis, vomiting, cough, flu syndrome, diarrhea, dysmenorrhea, fever, insomnia, and dyspepsia. **Infrequent:** Constipation, tremor, anxiety, pruritis, and vaginitis.

ADVERSE REACTIONS/TOXIC
WARNING: Potentially life-threatening rashes have been reported in association with the use of Lamotrigine. The rashes occur in approximately 1 in 1,000 adults.

NURSING MEASURES
1. Review history of seizure disorder (type, onset, intensity, frequency, duration, and level of consciousness).
2. Identify what prescription and over-the-counter medications the client is taking.
3. Identify amount and frequency of alcohol intake. Identify any other recreational drugs client is taking.

4. Identify other medical conditions, particularly renal or hepatic impairment.
5. Obtain baseline vital signs.
6. Report promptly any rash. May herald a life-threatening medical event.
7. Assess for dizziness or ataxia, and provide safety measures.
8. Assess for clinical improvement (decrease in intensity/frequency of seizures).

INFORM CLIENT AND FAMILY
1. Prior to initiation of treatment with Lamotrigine, the client and family should be instructed that a rash or other signs or symptoms of hypersensitivity (e.g., fever, lymphadenopathy, facial swelling) may herald a serious medical event. The client should report any such occurrence to a physician **immediately.**
2. Report first signs of a rash to the physician.
3. Antiepileptic drugs should not be abruptly discontinued because of the possibility of increasing seizure frequency, unless safety concerns (rash) require a rapid withdrawal.
4. Carry identification card; wear bracelet to note anticonvulsant therapy.
5. Avoid alcohol, lowers seizure threshold.

QUETIAPINE
(Seroquel)

ANTIPSYCHOTIC (DIBENZOTHIAZEPINE DERIVATIVE)

USES
Management of the manifestation of both positive and negative symptoms of schizophrenia.

ACTION
Interacts with multiple neurotransmitter receptors, including serotonin, dopamine, and histamine. Exact mechanism is unknown.

DOSAGES & ROUTES
PO Tablets (25 mg, 100 mg, or 200 mg)

Adult Initially 25 mg 2 times/day, then 25–50 mg a day up to a target dose of 300 mg/day given BID within 4–7days.

Elderly Because plasma clearance is reduced by 30–50% in elderly individuals, the rate of dose titration may need to be slower, and the daily therapeutic target dose lower.

CONTRAINDICATIONS
Quetiapine is contraindicated in people with a known hypersensitivity to this medication or any of its ingredients.

REMARKS
Precautions should be taken when using quetiapine in clients with preexisting hepatic disorders, in clients who are being treated with potentially hepatotoxic drugs, or if treatment-emergent signs or symptoms of hepatic impairment appear. Perform periodic liver function test.

SIDE EFFECTS
Frequent: Headache, somnolence, postural hypotension, dizziness, tachycardia, agitation, insomnia, dry mouth. May cause sedation and impair motor skills during initial dose titration period. **Infrequent**: Back pain, fever, and palpitation, weight gain, hyperthyroidism, rhinitis, leukopenia, ear pain.

ADVERSE REACTIONS
Cardiac: Elevated SGOT level. **Hepatic**: Elevated ALT (SGPT) levels. **Hematological:** Leukopenia. **Hormonal:** Reduction of thyroxin level usually during first 2–4 weeks of treatment.

NURSING MEASURES
1. Always monitor clients on antipsychotics for signs of:
   a. Tardive dyskinesia (TD)
   b. Neuoleptic malignant syndrome (NMS)
2. Assess for orthostatic hypotension, dizziness, and possible syncope during initial dose titration. Take necessary measures to prevent injury.
3. If client has a history of seizures or a condition associated with lowered seizure threshold, take necessary precautions.
4. For clients who have a known or suspected abnormal hepatic function or clients who develop any signs or symptoms suggestive of new onset liver disorder during quetiapine therapy, initial assessment and then periodic clinical assessment with thranaminase levels is recommended.

INFORM CLIENT AND FAMILY
1. Teach clients to inform their physician if they:
   a. Are about to become pregnant.
   b. Are breast feeding a baby.
   c. About over-the-counter and any prescription drugs they are taking (especially antihypertensive drugs).
   d. About any and all alcohol and recreational drug consumption.
2. To dangle feet before getting out of bed to prevent dizziness.
3. Since drug may slow cognitive function and motor skills initially, inform client to refrain from performing activities requiring mental alertness (driving, using hazardous machinery) until it is certain that the drug does not adversely affect their cognitive function.
4. Avoid alcohol while taking quetiapine since the cognitive and motor effects of alcohol consumption are potentiated with quetiapine.

REFERENCES

REFERENCES

Dubin, W.R., and Weiss, K.J. (1991). *Handbook of psychiatric emergencies*. Springhouse, PA: Springhouse Corporation.

Hodgson, B.B., Kizior, R.J., and Kindon, R.T. (1997). *Nurse's drug handbook 1997*. Philadelphia: W.B. Saunders Company.

Kaplan, H.I., and Sadock, B.J. (1993). *Pocket handbook of emergency psychiatric medicine*. Baltimore, MD: Williams & Wilkins.

Lehne, R.A., Moore, L.A., Crosby, L.J., et al. (1994). *Pharmacology for Nursing Care*, 2nd ed. Philadelphia: W.B. Saunders Company.

Slaby, A.E. (1994). *Handbook of psychiatric emergencies*, 4th ed. Norwalk, Connecticut: Appleton & Lange.

Schultz, J.M., and Dark, S.L. (1982). *Manual of psychiatric nursing care plans*. Boston: Little, Brown and Company.

Varcarolis, E.M. (1998). *Psychiatric mental health nursing*, 3rd ed. Philadelphia: W.B. Saunders Company.

Zuckerman, E.L. (1995). *Clinician's thesaurus*, 4th ed. New York: The Guilford Press.